# MEDICAL RESEARCH PROPOSAL, PAPER, AND THESIS WRITING

Xu-Feng Huang, MD, PhD, DSc
*Distinguished Professor of Medical Science*

Illawarra Health and Medical Research Institute
School of Medical, Indigenous and Health Sciences,
The University of Wollongong
Australia

2022



**Ashahi-Maple**

National Library of Australia Cataloguing-in-Publication Data is available.

First published in Australia in 2022

by Ashahi-Maple©, Inc.

ISBN 978-0-6454760-2-6

**TO MY FAMILY**

# Preface

Are you in the medical field, aiming to master research writing? This book is your comprehensive guide.

Key features include:

- Steps for preparing research proposals, papers, and high-degree theses.
- Tactics for effective literature searches.
- Tips on crafting abstracts, posters, tables, and figures.
- Techniques for honing your writing, from sentence structure to word choice.
- Special advice for beginners in medical research writing.
- Exemplary writings to guide and inspire your work.

Embark on your journey towards excellence in medical research writing and make a mark in healthcare and research with this essential manual.

Dr. Xu-Feng Huang, MD, PhD, DSc

# Contents

# PART ONE

# Research Proposal

## CHAPTER 1

A medical research proposal is a comprehensive document that outlines the plan and objectives for a proposed medical research study. It serves as a blueprint for conducting the research and seeks to convince relevant authorities, such as funding agencies, academic institutions, or ethics committees, of the significance and feasibility of the proposed investigation.

### Overview

### What should a medical proposal be about?

The medical research proposal should focus on a unique research question or hypothesis within your chosen field that is relevant, timely, and interesting to the medical community. You should seek to address a gap in current knowledge, provide new insights into a disease, medical condition, or healthcare practice, or propose a novel method or intervention that could potentially improve patient care.

The proposal ought to precisely elucidate the projected research concept or query and forecast the expected outcomes. The questions presented should lend a glimpse into the probable results while also defining the target beneficiaries of the study. This raises the fundamental question, "Who will benefit from the fruits of my research, and why is this study crucial?" Putting forth a captivating idea, projecting confidence grounded in existing research findings, and guaranteeing unequivocal clarity in your exposition is paramount.

Moreover, the proposal should lucidly elucidate the criticality of the project's aims and delineate the strategies employed to accomplish these objectives. The research design is key and should be tailored to address and provide answers to the research questions.

Ultimately, the proposal must assert the significance of the research idea and its value to the medical field. This involves demonstrating how it will enhance knowledge, improve patient care, or inform health policy.

Furthermore, your research proposal should clearly explain what you plan to do and demonstrate your understanding of the topic, your ability to conduct the research, and your consideration of your work's ethical and practical implications. It's also beneficial to show how your work will contribute to the existing body of knowledge.

## Research proposal writing guidelines

General guidelines for preparing biomedical, medical, exercise, or nutrition research proposal

A research proposal is a comprehensive plan that outlines a research study's objectives, methods, and potential impact. Whether it's biomedical, medical, exercise, or nutrition research, a well-structured proposal is essential to secure funding, gain ethical approval, and ensure the study's success.

Below are general guidelines to consider when creating a research proposal in these fields:

1. **Title**: The title should be concise and accurately reflect the research content.
2. **Background/Literature Review**: Present the background information and summarize relevant studies to provide the context and justification for your research. This section should highlight the knowledge gap your research will fill.
3. **Aims/Objectives**: Clearly state the aims and objectives of your research. These should be SMART - Specific, Measurable, Achievable, Relevant, and Time-bound.
4. **Research Question/Hypothesis**: State the research question or hypothesis that your project will address. Ensure that it is clear, focused, and answerable.
5. **Methods**: Detail the methodologies that you will use in the research. This should include study design, data collection methods, data analysis techniques, and any software or equipment you use. Be sure to justify your choice of methods.

   **Study Population**: Describe the population from which you'll draw your sample, the sample size, and how participants will be selected.

   **Ethical Considerations**: Discuss any ethical issues arising during the research and how you plan to address them. For medical or health-related research, consider issues like informed consent, confidentiality, and the handling of personal data.

**Timeline**: Include a timeline that outlines the different phases of your research, from data collection to analysis and writing up.

**Budget**: Provide a detailed budget outlining how funds will be used if necessary. It should cover equipment, participant compensation, software, and travel expenses.

**Impact and Significance**: Explain the potential impact of your research and its significance to your field. How will it contribute to current knowledge or practices? How could it potentially influence policy or affect health outcomes?

**Limitations**: Address potential limitations of your research, and how you plan to minimize their impact.

6. **References**: Cite all sources that you have referred to in your proposal.

Note: Different research proposals may require specific additional sections or modifications based on the scope and nature of the study. In practice, each section would be further elaborated and expanded upon in the actual proposal document to provide sufficient detail and clarity. Always follow the guidelines provided by the funding agency or institution and seek feedback from mentors or colleagues to refine and strengthen your research proposal before submission.

## Emphases of a research proposal

When preparing a proposal, the topic, justification, and approach should be emphasized. It is a good idea to keep in mind that the emphasis should be in a way that aligns with the expectations and priorities of your audience, which could include funding agencies, institutional review boards, or other researchers in your field. Different audiences may place more or less emphasis on various elements, so it's essential to understand their needs and tailor your proposal accordingly.

**How long should a proposal be?**

The length of a research proposal can vary significantly depending on the institution's requirements or the funding body you are submitting. However, a general guideline is that a research proposal should be between 1,500 and 3,000 words, or around 3 to 6 pages if the proposal is single-spaced and twice if it is double-spaced.

In some cases, such as for Ph.D. applications, a research proposal might be more extended, perhaps up to 10,000 words. Conversely, if you are applying for specific funding or grants, you may be asked to submit a shorter proposal or a particular outline.

Regardless of length, your proposal should be clear and concise and provide sufficient detail to allow the reader to understand your research question, why it's important, and how you plan to answer it.

Always check the specific requirements of the institution or body to which you are submitting your proposal, as they may have specific guidelines on length and format. Failure to adhere to these could result in your proposal being rejected, regardless of the quality of your research idea.

## Title

Constructing an excellent proposal title in research is crucial as it serves as the first impression of your research project. A well-crafted title should be concise, informative, and engaging, effectively conveying the essence of your research.

Practically, you could consider the following: what the project is doing, how it does, where to perform the task, and for whom. Try to describe the value of the project, but don't be too descriptive, and keep it simple, clear, and understandable without explanation. Try to use a combination of a subject, verb, and object.

Not "Helping Diabetes Patients." This title is vague because it does not say how to help and who will benefit. Instead, you could say, "Encouraging Moderate Exercise Improves Insulin Resistance in Elderly Diabetes Patients in City A."

**Here are some tips to help you create a proposal title:**

- **Be Clear and Specific:** Your title should reflect the main focus of your research. Avoid vague or overly broad titles that might not convey the exact purpose of the study. Instead, include specific keywords that highlight the subject and scope of your research.
- **Highlight the Key Variables or Interventions:** If your research involves specific variables or interventions, include them in the title. This will give readers an immediate understanding of the main factors being studied.
- **Consider the Study Design:** If your research follows a particular study design, such as a randomized controlled

trial, meta-analysis, or cohort study, consider incorporating it into the title. This adds valuable information and context to your proposal.

- **Be Engaging and Captivating:** While maintaining clarity, try to make the title engaging and captivating. A well-crafted title can generate interest in your research and entice readers to explore further.
- **Mention the Target Population:** If your study focuses on a specific population or patient group, include that information in the title. This will help readers understand the relevance and applicability of your research.
- **Keep it Concise:** Keep your title concise and to the point. Ideally, a title should be no longer than 15 words. Short titles are more memorable and easier to comprehend.
- **Use Precise Language:** Choose precise and straightforward language in your title. Avoid jargon or acronyms that may not be familiar to all readers. Aim for clarity and readability.
- **Avoid Abbreviations**: Generally, it's best to avoid abbreviations in the title. Spell out important terms to ensure clarity and avoid confusion.
- **Review Existing Literature:** Before finalizing your title, search for similar studies in the existing literature. Ensure that your title stands out and doesn't closely resemble others in the field.
- **Seek Feedback:** After drafting your title, seek feedback from colleagues or mentors in the medical or research community. They can offer valuable insights and suggestions for improvement.

### Project Supervisor

Provide the name, qualification, and school of the academic institution. It is suggested that you work with your research supervisor to define the proposed research and ensure it meets the requirements of the degree of your study.

### Abstract

All proposals should have an abstract. An abstract should present the whole story of the proposal. By reading the abstract, the reviewer can understand the basics of the project. Therefore, the reader should not have to rely on reading other parts of the document to understand the basics of the project. Usually, reviewers read the abstract first and again last. Therefore, you could lose the reviewer's interest in reading your proposal if you have written a poor abstract. Thus, the abstract is the most important single part of the proposal.

### What should you write in the abstract?

Overall, an abstract should present the meaning of the proposal. You can start with the project's motivation; provide the hypothesis, main objectives, and procedures to be carried out to accomplish the goals; and summarize the significance and potential impact of the work.

*What are the essential components of a research proposal?*

A research proposal abstract typically summarizes the main aspects of the entire proposal in a condensed form. Writing an abstract can be challenging, as it needs to be concise yet highly informative. Here are the essential components of a research proposal abstract:

- **Background/Introduction:** Briefly mention the broader context and importance of the research problem you are planning to address. State the significance of the research, explaining why it's important and who it benefits.
- **Objective/Purpose:** Clearly state your research's objective or primary purpose. What are you aiming to achieve or find out with your research?
- **Research Question/Hypothesis:** State the specific question(s) or hypothesis your research intends to answer or investigate. These should be precise and succinct.
- **Methodology:** Briefly describe the methods you plan to use to conduct your research. This might include your study design, data collection, and analysis methods.
- **Expected Results/Implications**: Indicate the expected outcomes and how they will contribute to the field of study. Explain how your results could possibly impact future research, policy, or practice.

Remember that an abstract should be brief (usually around 250 words, depending on the guidelines) and clearly articulate each component. Avoid going into unnecessary detail, and don't include any citations in the abstract.

## Table of Contents

The table of contents is the roadmap indicating the components of your proposal. It provides an overview of the proposal and lets reviewers find the sections of their interest. It can also help reviewers navigate and understand the text while reading. A table of contents lists what the proposal includes. The list can be chapter titles and section titles together with page numbers.

## Literature Review

Writing a literature review for a research proposal involves summarizing and evaluating the current knowledge on a specific topic from credible sources. Here is a step-by-step guide:

1. **Understand Your Topic**: You need to understand the area you are researching. What are the key issues, debates, theories, or concepts? How has the field developed over time? What gaps still exist in our understanding?

2. **Search for Relevant Literature**: This will primarily involve academic papers, books, articles, reports, etc. Depending on your field, you can use academic databases like Google Scholar, PubMed, and Web of Science. Remember to focus on the most relevant and recent sources to stay up-to-date.

3. **Critical Appraisal**: Don't just take the authors' words for it - evaluate the validity and reliability of the work. Consider the methodology, data, analysis, and conclusions.

4. **Take Notes**: As you read, take notes. These should not just be descriptive but also analytical. Write down key arguments, methods, findings, and thoughts about the work.
5. **Categorize Your Sources**: This could be methodology, theme, chronology, sector, etc. This will help in synthesizing the literature later.
6. **Write the Review**:
   - **Introduction**: Here, you introduce the topic and your research question. You also need to state the objectives of the literature review.
   - **Body**: This is where you discuss the literature. You may want to structure your body accordingly depending on how you've categorized your sources. Summarizing each category's significant findings, debates, and gaps would be best. Remember to compare and contrast different authors' views, discuss areas of controversy, and show patterns or trends in the literature.
   - **Conclusion**: Summarize the significant contributions, debates, and gaps in the literature. Based on this, justify your research. Your research proposal should address a gap or take a novel approach.
7. **Reference List**: Finally, you should provide a list of all sources you've cited in your literature review, formatted according to your specified citation style (APA, MLA, Chicago, etc.)

Remember, a literature review is not just about describing what others have found, but about identifying patterns, gaps, or debates in the literature and positioning your own research within this context.

## Emphases:

*Problem or question:* Try to use a couple of precise sentences detailing the essentials of the current state of the problem and the significance of solving the problem. You should explain why the proposed work is necessary and requires an answer. It will help if you use previous research to justify the proposed research and tell what we know and what we do not know. Keep in mind that all information used must be relevant to the investigations.

*Originality:* The literature review should be selective, aiming toward research originality and innovation, which require accurate and in-depth justification. In this regard, you need to provide sufficient information to explain the ingenuity or creativity of the proposed work.

*Significance:* Why is this research needed? How would the outcomes of the proposed research fill this need? What are the benefits?

## To present a research gap

State how your research will contribute to the existing literature in the field: Think of the things that were not explored by previous studies. Then, write how your research tackles those unexplored areas. Through this, you can convince your readers that you are studying something new and adding value to the field.

You should identify the research gap in the introductory or literature review section. Based on existing studies, you may clearly outline what is currently known about the topic and then identify where the gaps in knowledge or understanding lie. This could be a question that hasn't been answered, a theory that hasn't been tested, or a population or context that hasn't been studied.

A research gap is where no or limited research has been conducted. It's essentially a missing piece in the current body of knowledge about a particular subject. Identifying and addressing these gaps is a fundamental part of research, as it helps to advance our understanding of the field.

Your research question or hypothesis should be directly related to this gap, and your proposed study should aim to fill it. By doing this, you demonstrate the relevance and significance of your research and justify why it should be conducted.

Let's say you're writing a proposal about diabetes management. If existing research has focused on adults, but little is known about diabetes management in adolescents, this would represent a research gap. Your research question could be something like, "What are the most effective strategies for managing diabetes in adolescents?" and your study could aim to answer this question.

Remember that identifying a research gap requires thoroughly reviewing the existing literature on your topic. This helps to ensure that the gap you've identified is genuine and that your research will make a meaningful contribution to your field.

## Hypothesis, Aims, and Objectives

Formulating a research hypothesis is a crucial step in the scientific process as it lays the foundation for the research design. A hypothesis is a statement that predicts the relationship between two or more variables.

Here is a step-by-step approach to construct a hypothesis for a research proposal:

1. **Identify your research question**: Before you start formulating a hypothesis, you must have a specific research question. This research question is often driven by the broader research problem that you aim to address. For example, the question might be, "Does regular exercise affect mental health?" The question identifies two variables - regular exercise (independent variable) and mental health (dependent variable).
2. **Do a Literature Review**: Research what has already been done in the field regarding your question. This will give you an understanding of the theoretical framework and help you predict the potential outcomes of your research. This can help in formulating your hypothesis.
3. **Formulate your Hypothesis**: Based on your research question and literature review, you can formulate your hypothesis. A hypothesis is a predictive statement about the relationship between two or more variables. For the given

example, the hypothesis might be, "Regular exercise leads to improved mental health."

4. **Ensure Your Hypothesis is Testable**: It's crucial that your hypothesis can be tested through empirical research methods. A testable hypothesis is one that can be supported or refuted through experimentation or more generally, empirical evidence. For our example, you can design a study where one group of participants engages in regular exercise and another does not, and then you measure their mental health to see if there's a significant difference.

5. **Keep your Hypothesis Specific and Simple**: A good hypothesis is one that is simple and specific. It should clearly define the relationship between the variables and should be straightforward enough that anyone reading it would understand what you plan to research.

6. **Formulate Null and Alternative Hypotheses**: In many statistical tests, you'll need to formulate a null hypothesis (which proposes that there is no significant relationship between the variables) and an alternative hypothesis (which proposes there is a significant relationship). In our example, the null hypothesis would be "Regular exercise does not affect mental health," while the alternative hypothesis would be "Regular exercise improves mental health."

7. **Revise and Refine**: Finally, once you've formulated your hypothesis, take the time to revise and refine it. This might involve peer review, where other experts in your field review your hypothesis and provide feedback. Through this process, you can refine your hypothesis to ensure that it is

not only testable but also relevant and significant to your field.

8. Remember that a hypothesis is not set in stone. It can be revised or discarded if the research data does not support it. But a well-constructed hypothesis can provide a strong guide for your research design and analysis.

**Similarity and differences between the hypothesis, aim and objectives.**

The hypothesis, aim, and objective are essential components of a research proposal, and each serves a different function. Understanding the similarities and differences can help you structure your research more effectively.

1. **Hypothesis**

A hypothesis is a predictive statement about the potential outcome of the research, usually asserting a relationship between two or more variables. It's a tentative explanation for an observation, phenomenon, or scientific problem that can be tested by further investigation.

Similarity: Like aims and objectives, a hypothesis is future-oriented and relates to what you hope to achieve or discover in your research.

Difference: Unlike aims and objectives, a hypothesis is often presented as a statement that can be proven true or false. It is generally tested through various research methods and directly contributes to the development of theoretical knowledge. It's specific and testable, often positing a relationship between variables.

2. **Aim**

The aim of a study is a broad statement indicating the goals or purpose of the research. It outlines what the researcher wants to achieve at the end of the research project.

Similarity: Like a hypothesis and objectives, the aim is future-oriented and guides the direction of the research.

Difference: The aim of a study is broader and less specific than a hypothesis or objectives. While a hypothesis makes a specific prediction that can be tested, and objectives outline specific steps to be taken, the aim gives a general direction for the research.

3. **Objectives**

Objectives are specific, measurable steps that a researcher plans to take to achieve the research aim. They are more precise and detailed than the aim, often presented as actionable items.

Similarity: Like aims and hypotheses, objectives relate to what you hope to achieve in your research.

Difference: Objectives are usually more detailed and concrete than the aim or hypothesis. They are the specific steps you will take to achieve your aim and guide your methodology. Unlike a hypothesis, objectives are not typically concerned with predicting the outcome of the research; instead, they define the path to reach the aim.

In summary, the hypothesis, aim, and objectives are essential components of a research study, each with a unique role. The hypothesis provides a *specific prediction to be tested*, the aim gives the research its *overarching purpose*, and the objectives outline the *specific steps* to reach that purpose.

## Methods

The Methods section, also known as the Methodology or Research Design section, is a key component of a research proposal. This section provides a detailed account of the steps that you plan to take to achieve your research objectives. While the specifics may vary slightly depending on your field of study and the nature of your research, the following components are typically included in the Methods section of a research proposal:

1. **Research Design**: This involves clearly explaining the type of research you will be conducting. This could be experimental, observational, or another type. It also involves describing the overall structure of the research process.
2. **Participants/Subjects**: Describe who will participate in your research (e.g., people, organizations, animals, cells, etc.), including how they will be selected, recruited, and assigned to different groups if necessary.

3. **Data Collection Procedures**: Discuss the specific methods you will use to gather your data. This could include surveys, interviews, observations, etc. You need to provide enough detail so that others can replicate your methods.
4. **Materials:** The materials are what you use in your research. These include your experiments' raw materials, equipment, and chemicals.
5. **Instruments**: Describe any tools or devices used in your study, such as questionnaires, tests, or laboratory equipment. Consider providing a few example questions if you're using a survey or questionnaire.
6. **Data Analysis**: Discuss the techniques you'll use to process and analyze the data you collect. This could include statistical tests, coding methods for qualitative data, or methods for interpreting experimental results.
7. **Ethical Considerations**: Address any ethical issues related to your research. This might involve a discussion of informed consent, confidentiality, potential risks to participants, and how these risks will be mitigated.
8. **Validity and Reliability**: Explain how you'll ensure your results are reliable (consistent results if the study were to be replicated) and valid (accurately representing what they're supposed to represent).
9. **Limitations:** Discuss potential weaknesses or limitations of your proposed study and methods. This shows reviewers that you're aware of these issues and have thought about how to handle them.

10. **Timeframe:** Include an estimated timeline for your project. This should include the time needed for each stage of the research process. A timeline is part of the research plan. In the timeline, you may itemize the list of deliverables with specific dates so you can make efforts to achieve the tasks.

    The graphic below is an example timeline of a three-year research project. There are many ways to make timeline indicators. You may also refer to the institution's guidelines.

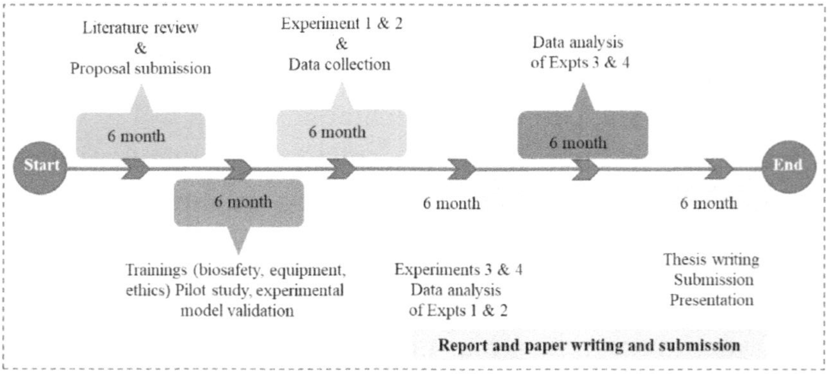


## Expected Outcomes

The expected outcomes of a research proposal are the results you anticipate from the research project. These should be realistic, clearly articulated, and tied directly to the goals and objectives of the project. Here are some tips on how to write the expected outcomes:

1. **Clearly Define Your Objectives**: Expected outcomes should relate directly to the objectives of the research. State

your objectives clearly and then explain how the expected outcomes address these objectives.

2. **Be Specific**: Your outcomes should be specific and detailed, explaining what you expect to discover or confirm through your research. Avoid vague or general statements.
3. **Quantify Where Possible**: If your research involves the analysis of statistical data, be clear about what results you expect. Include specific numbers, percentages, or ranges whenever possible.
4. **Use Actionable Language**: Make sure that your outcomes can be directly acted upon. Use verbs that indicate action, such as "increase," "reduce," "identify," "determine," etc.
5. **Make them Measurable**: Outcomes should be measurable so you can determine if you've reached them at the end of your research. They need to be realistic and achievable given your resources and time frame.
6. **Explain the Relevance**: Explain why these outcomes are relevant. In what way do they contribute to existing medical knowledge? How can they be applied in practice?

## Significance

The significance section of a medical research proposal is a critical component where you must demonstrate your study's relevance and potential impact. It also helps the reader understand why your research topic should be given priority and funding.

The key to writing an effective significance section is clearly articulating how your research will advance knowledge in your field and contribute to better health outcomes or understanding disease processes.

Here are steps to write a compelling significance section:

1. **Identify the Gap in Current Knowledge or Practice:** This is the first step in writing the significance of a research proposal. Show how your research fills a critical gap in current knowledge or practice in your field. Describe how addressing this gap can lead to important new insights, treatments, or understanding.
2. **State the Importance of Your Research Topic:** Clearly state why your topic is important. You can do this by highlighting the prevalence or severity of the problem you're studying, its relevance to human health, and/or its potential to advance the medical field.
3. **Describe the Potential Impact of Your Research:** Explain how your research will contribute to current knowledge or practice. This can include new methodologies, theories, treatments, or understanding. Also, consider the broader implications, such as potential changes in healthcare policies, clinical guidelines, or preventive strategies.
4. **Relate to Broader Societal Implications:** Emphasize how your research will affect society. This can include reducing healthcare costs, improving patient outcomes, increasing the understanding of disease mechanisms, or addressing health disparities.

5. **Highlight Innovation:** Point out how your research is innovative. This can mean applying new methodologies, exploring uncharted territories in your field, or bringing together disciplines in novel ways.
6. **Indicate the Sustainability of Your Research:** Show that your research can lead to further studies and has the potential for long-term impact.

## Validity of the research plan

Explain how your research will benefit society. In this part, tell how your research will impact society. Think of how the results of your research will change something in your community.

Addressing validity in your research proposal is essential to ensure the reliability of your results and the strength of your conclusions. There are different types of validity to consider:

**Internal Validity:** This refers to the degree to which the results of your study can be attributed to your independent variable(s) and not some other factor. You can increase internal validity by controlling confounding variables, randomizing your sample, and employing a good experimental design.

**External Validity:** This refers to the extent to which the results of your study can be generalized to other contexts, settings, or populations. You can increase external validity by using a representative sample and ensuring the conditions of your study mimic real-world situations as closely as possible.

**Construct Validity:** This is the extent to which your measures accurately represent the concept you are studying. To increase construct validity, you might use validated measurement instruments to clearly define and operationalize your variables.

**Content Validity:** This refers to how well your measure covers the entire range of the concept's meaning. To increase content validity, the research should cover all aspects of the concept you're researching.

**Criterion-related Validity:** This measures how a variable or set of variables predicts an outcome based on a criterion or set of criteria. It is divided into concurrent and predictive validity.

In your proposal, you should explain your strategies to maximize the validity of your study. This could involve careful selection and operationalization of your variables, research design and methodology choice, data collection methods, statistical analysis, etc.

It's important to remember that no study is perfectly valid. There will always be limitations that could potentially impact validity. Be upfront about these in your proposal and discuss how you plan to minimize their impact. This demonstrates your understanding of the research process and increases the trustworthiness of your proposal.

## References

Here is what a reference list in a research proposal should cover:

1. **Completeness**: The reference list should include all the sources you've cited in the proposal. If you've mentioned a

study, theory, or academic contribution in your proposal, it should appear in the reference list.

2. **Relevance**: The sources you cite should be relevant to your research question and contribute to constructing your proposal's rationale or methodology. The reference list isn't the place to show off everything you've read on the topic – only include the most relevant and significant sources that directly support your proposed research.
3. **Currency**: In some fields, it's important to cite recent sources to show that you are up-to-date with the latest research. However, seminal works of key theorists in the field should also be included, even if they are older.
4. **Authoritative Sources**: Ensure the sources you reference are credible and authoritative. These are usually peer-reviewed articles or published books. Be cautious when citing sources such as blogs or websites without a rigorous review process.
5. **Cross-checking**: Make sure that in-text citations and the reference list entries correspond to each other, with no extra sources in either place.

In essence, a reference list provides the validation of your literature review and demonstrates your capacity to join the scholarly conversation on your chosen topic.

## Reference management software

Reference management software can significantly simplify the process of organizing and formatting citations and bibliographies in research proposals. Here are some of the most commonly used tools in the medical field:

1. **EndNote**: This is a widely used reference management software in various disciplines, including medicine. It allows you to collect and organize references and format bibliographies in thousands of citation styles.
2. **Mendeley**: Mendeley is another popular choice among medical researchers. It allows you to store, organize, and format your references. It also includes a social networking aspect where you can collaborate with other researchers.
3. **Zotero**: Zotero is a free, open-source software that helps you collect, organize, cite, and share research. It's compatible with a wide variety of browsers and word processors.
4. **RefWorks**: This cloud-based software is used for reference management, including document and citation sharing. It's used in many fields, including medical research.

The choice among these software options often depends on personal preference, the project's specific needs, the research team's size, and the available budget (since some tools require a paid subscription). Always consider these factors when choosing reference management software.

## Proposal Template

| Research Proposal Template | |
|---|---|
| Project title | |
| Candidate's name | |
| Supervisor's name | |
| Organization | |
| Year | |
| 1. ABSTRACT (250–500 words) | |
| Research Motivation<br>Justification or rationale of the project<br>Hypothesis, aim, and objectives<br>Research Methods<br>Expected outcomes and significance | |
| 2. LIST OF CONTENTS (1–2 pages) | |
| Develop a table of contents indicating the page numbers of each chapter. | |
| 3. LITERATURE REVIEW<br>Research question, research field, study justification, aims, and significance (5–6 pages) | |
| Raise a research question and determine the keywords.<br>Decide on search engines or databases to be used.<br>Find and evaluate relevant papers.<br>Synthesize and analyze the data from papers.<br>Provide research justifications and significance. | |
| 4. HYPOTHESIS, AIM, AND OBJECTIVES (0.5 pages) | |
| Relate to the research question.<br>Define the independent and dependent variables.<br>Make sure it is testable. | |
| 5. METHODS (3-5 pages) | |

| |
|---|
| Research design, variables, groups, duration, measurements Data collection, Statistical analysis, etc. |
| EXPECTED OUTCOMES AND SIGNIFICANCE (0.5–1 page) |
| List what you expect to achieve at the end of the study. Explain the desired impact and benefit of the proposed research. |
| REFERENCES<br>Provide a list of the papers cited in the proposal. |

**Examples**

## Clinical Proposal Title Example 1

*"Long-Term Effects of Mediterranean Diet on Cognitive Function in Elderly Individuals: A Prospective Cohort Study"* Explanation: This title clearly states the main focus of the research (Mediterranean Diet and Cognitive Function), the target population (Elderly Individuals), and the study design (Prospective Cohort Study). It highlights the potential benefits of the Mediterranean diet on cognitive health in aging, making it an engaging and relevant title.

## Clinical Proposal Title Example 2

*"Exploring the Impact of Social Engagement on Loneliness and Mental Health among Aging Adults: A Cross-Sectional Analysis"* Explanation: This title addresses an important aspect of aging research (Social Engagement, Loneliness, and Mental Health),

and the study design (Cross-Sectional Analysis) is mentioned. It hints at potential insights into how social interactions affect mental well-being in the elderly, making it an intriguing and meaningful title.

**Clinical Proposal Title Example 3**

*"Effect of Regular Physical Activity on Mobility and Independence in Older Adults: A Randomized Intervention Trial"* Explanation: This title focuses on the intervention (Regular Physical Activity) and its potential benefits on aging-related outcomes (Mobility and Independence). The mention of the study design (Randomized Intervention Trial) adds credibility and interest to the proposal.

**Clinical Proposal Title Example 4**

*"Unraveling the Genetic Determinants of Longevity: A Genome-Wide Association Study in a Geriatric Population"* Explanation: This title highlights the research objective (Genetic Determinants of Longevity) and the study approach (Genome-Wide Association Study). It indicates the use of cutting-edge genomic methods to explore factors contributing to longevity in the elderly, making it an innovative and scientifically significant title.

**Clinical Proposal Title Example 5**

*"Assessing the Impact of Sleep Quality on Cognitive Decline in Aging: A Longitudinal Analysis"* Explanation: The title clearly states the main variables under investigation (Sleep Quality

and Cognitive Decline) and the study design (Longitudinal Analysis). It suggests a comprehensive examination of the relationship between sleep and cognitive health over time, making it an important and well-defined title.

**Clinical Proposal Title Example 6**

*"A Multimodal Approach to Understanding Brain Aging: Neuroimaging, Cognitive Assessment, and Biomarker Analysis"* Explanation: This title indicates the utilization of a multidimensional approach (Neuroimaging, Cognitive Assessment, and Biomarker Analysis) to study brain aging. It highlights the comprehensive nature of the research, making it a compelling and well-rounded title.

**Preclinical Proposal Title Example 1**

*"Neuroprotective Effects of Curcumin in a Rat Model of Alzheimer's Disease: A Histopathological and Behavioral Analysis"* Explanation: This title is excellent because it clearly indicates the main focus of the study (Neuroprotective Effects of Curcumin), the target model (Rat Model of Alzheimer's Disease), and the methodology (Histopathological and Behavioral Analysis). It promises valuable insights into the potential therapeutic benefits of curcumin for Alzheimer's disease, and it includes key variables and interventions.

**Preclinical Proposal Title Example 2**

*"Assessment of Novel Drug Delivery System for Targeted Chemotherapy in Triple-Negative Breast Cancer Xenografts"*

Explanation: This title is strong because it highlights the purpose of the study (Assessment of Novel Drug Delivery System) and its specific application (Targeted Chemotherapy) in a particular cancer type (Triple-Negative Breast Cancer Xenografts). It informs readers about the innovative aspect of the research and its potential clinical implications.

**Preclinical Proposal Title Example 3**

*"Investigating the Immunomodulatory Effects of Mesenchymal Stem Cells in a Mouse Model of Inflammatory Bowel Disease"* Explanation: This title is effective because it conveys the main objective (Investigating the Immunomodulatory Effects) and the intervention being studied (Mesenchymal Stem Cells) in the context of a specific disease model (Mouse Model of Inflammatory Bowel Disease). It showcases the relevance of the research to potential therapeutic approaches for inflammatory bowel disease.

**Preclinical Proposal Title Example 4**

*"Effects of a Hydrogel Scaffold on Cartilage Regeneration in a Rabbit Model of Osteoarthritis"* Explanation: This title is strong because it highlights the central focus (Effects of a Hydrogel Scaffold), the outcome of interest (Cartilage Regeneration), and the disease model used (Rabbit Model of Osteoarthritis). It clearly conveys the potential application of the hydrogel scaffold for osteoarthritis treatment.

The proposal titles are clear, specific, and concise in each of these examples. They effectively convey the main objective, the specific intervention or variables being studied, and the disease models used. Additionally, they provide enough information to generate interest and showcase the potential significance of the research, making them excellent proposal titles for preclinical research.

## Abstract Example 1

*"Effectiveness of Mediterranean Diet in the Prevention of Type 2 Diabetes Among Prediabetic Individuals: A Randomized Controlled Trial"*

Abstract: This proposal aims to investigate the effectiveness of a Mediterranean diet in preventing the progression from prediabetes to Type 2 Diabetes (T2D). The study proposes a randomized controlled trial with a sample size of 1000 prediabetic adults divided into two groups - one following a Mediterranean diet and another following a standard diet - for three years. Primary outcome measures will include changes in glycated hemoglobin (HbA1c) levels and the conversion rate to T2D. It is hypothesized that adherence to a Mediterranean diet will result in improved glycemic control and reduced T2D incidence. Expected results could reinforce the role of dietary intervention in T2D prevention strategies and contribute to more effective dietetic guidelines for prediabetic individuals.

## Abstract Example 2

*"Investigating the Role of Aerobic Exercise in Enhancing Cognitive Health in Aging: A Research Proposal"*

Abstract: Cognitive health in aging populations is a growing concern, with potential links to lifestyle factors like physical activity remaining underexplored. This proposal examines aerobic exercise's impact on cognition using an aging model. The central hypothesis is that a consistent aerobic exercise regimen can mitigate age-related cognitive decline. The proposed methodology involves a combination of cognitive assessments and neuroimaging techniques to measure changes in cognitive function and brain structures over time. Anticipated results could significantly contribute to our understanding of exercise as a preventative strategy for cognitive decline, encouraging its incorporation into public health guidelines and aging care practices. Additionally, our research could pave the way for more in-depth investigations on the neurobiological mechanisms behind the cognitive benefits of aerobic exercise.

Pros: Specific mention of neuroimaging techniques signals a rigorous and objective methodology that could provide more reliable and convincing results. Highlights the research's potential to influence public health guidelines: This indicates the real-world implications of the findings.

Cons: Lacks explicit mention of qualitative interviews: Qualitative data could provide additional depth and context to the findings. Without mentioning it, the research might seem less comprehensive. Less explicit mention of the health issue at hand: While it does say that cognitive health in aging is a concern, it might be more impactful to directly address the issue of cognitive decline or dementia in the aging population.

**Abstract Example 3**

*Understanding the Preventive Mechanism of Butyrate in Obesity: A Preclinical Trial*

**Background/Introduction:** Obesity is a global health concern with significant morbidity and mortality, requiring novel preventative and therapeutic approaches. Recent evidence suggests butyrate, a short-chain fatty acid produced by gut microbiota, may be crucial in obesity prevention.

**Objective/Purpose:** This study aims to elucidate how butyrate exerts its anti-obesity effects, potentially paving the way for new preventive strategies against obesity.

**Research Question/Hypothesis:** We hypothesize that butyrate influences metabolic regulation, leading to obesity prevention. This research seeks to determine how butyrate modulates these metabolic pathways in a preclinical model.

**Methodology:** We will use a preclinical animal model to induce obesity conditions and administer butyrate in controlled dosages. Subsequent changes in metabolic pathways, body weight, fat accumulation, and gut microbiome composition will be examined through various assays, histological analysis, and next-generation sequencing.

**Expected Results/Implications:** We anticipate that butyrate administration will lead to decreased obesity indicators, thus establishing its potential as an obesity preventive measure. Our findings may offer critical insights into butyrate's mechanism of action and inspire new avenues for obesity prevention strategies.

You may combine the above content into a single paragraph within 250 words.

Obesity, a significant global health issue with high morbidity and mortality rates, demands innovative preventive and therapeutic strategies. Recently, attention has been drawn to the potential role of butyrate, a short-chain fatty acid produced by gut microbiota, in averting obesity. This research aims to unravel the mechanism through which butyrate inhibits obesity, thereby potentially facilitating the development of novel obesity prevention strategies. Our working hypothesis posits that butyrate might exert an influential role in regulating metabolic pathways, leading to obesity prevention. A preclinical animal model will be used to test this hypothesis. After inducing obesity conditions, we will introduce butyrate in controlled doses. The subsequent alterations in metabolic processes, body weight, fat accumulation, and gut microbiome composition will be scrutinized through various assays, histological analysis, and next-generation sequencing. We expect that butyrate administration will correlate with diminished obesity markers, thereby solidifying its potential role in obesity prevention. The anticipated findings from this research could shed crucial light on the metabolic mechanisms of butyrate action, thereby inspiring new directions in obesity prevention and treatment strategies.

## Literature Review Example 1

*"Dietary fiber for weight management: A randomized controlled trial."*

**Introduction:** The role of dietary fiber in weight management is a topic of intense research and public interest. Despite a multitude of studies, the relationship between dietary fiber intake and weight loss remains nuanced and complex. This review aims to critically examine the current body of literature on dietary fiber and weight management, focusing on randomized controlled trials (RCTs).

### Body

**Early Research and Basic Concepts:** The earliest studies related to dietary fiber and weight management focused primarily on the mechanical effects of fiber intake, suggesting that high fiber consumption could increase satiety and reduce energy intake (Refs). Similarly, the association between fiber intake and slower absorption of nutrients, leading to a more prolonged feeling of fullness, was reported (Ref).

**RCTs on Soluble and Insoluble Fibers:** More recent RCTs have endeavored to elucidate the differential effects of soluble and insoluble fibers on weight loss. A meta-analysis (Ref) found that soluble fibers had a small but significant effect on promoting weight loss in overweight individuals. In contrast, results for insoluble fibers were more variable, suggesting a more complex relationship, potentially influenced by other dietary factors (Ref). Despite these findings, the heterogeneity of studies in terms of fiber type, dosage, and duration of interventions adds complexity to conclusions (Refs).

**Fiber as a Component of a Healthy Diet:** Another trend in recent research is the examination of fiber as part of broader dietary patterns. Several large-scale observational studies and RCTs have associated higher fiber intakes with lower body weights in healthy dietary patterns, such as the Mediterranean diet (Ref) and DASH diet (Ref). However, whether fiber is a key driver of these effects or a marker of a generally healthy diet is still under debate.

**Gaps in Current Knowledge:** While existing research provides valuable insights, there remain critical gaps in our knowledge. Many studies have been of short duration and small sample size, limiting their external validity (Ref). There is a need for more high-quality, large-scale RCTs to explore the effects of different types of dietary fiber on weight management, especially in diverse populations. Additionally, understanding the interplay of dietary fiber with other dietary and lifestyle factors is paramount to forming coherent dietary guidelines.

**Conclusion:** The role of dietary fiber in weight management has been examined in numerous studies, offering promising yet complex results. The evidence suggests that while increasing fiber intake could contribute to weight loss, the overall diet's type of fiber and context may play significant roles. The proposed study will build on this body of research, addressing gaps by conducting a large-scale, long-term RCT examining the effects of specific types of dietary fiber on weight loss in a diverse population.

## References

(In this section, you would include all the works cited in the review, formatted according to the chosen citation style.)

**The below questions are for focused group discussions.**

1. **Methodological Differences**: Given the variability in results across studies due to differences in fiber type, dosage, and intervention duration, how could our study design ensure a more standardized approach that can yield more comparable results?
2. **Soluble vs. Insoluble Fiber**: Considering the findings from previous studies (refs) on soluble and insoluble fibers, should our study focus on one type of fiber over the other, or is there a need for a comparative study on the impact of both types on weight management?
3. **Fiber in the Context of a Healthy Diet**: As pointed out in the studies on the Mediterranean and DASH diets, fiber intake is often part of a broader healthy dietary pattern. How can our study design account for or control these potentially confounding factors?
4. **Population Diversity**: Since previous studies have often been critiqued for their lack of diversity, how can we ensure our study includes a broad, diverse population to enhance external validity?
5. **Practical Application**: How can the results of our study potentially influence dietary guidelines or recommendations, and what steps can we take to ensure

our results are presented in a way that is actionable for dietitians, clinicians, and the public?

These questions aim to provoke critical thinking about the proposed research and ensure it is designed to fill identified gaps in the existing literature.

### Literature Review Example 2

*"Microglia on brain ageing: a preclinical study"*

**Introduction:** The impact of aging on the human brain has been the focus of extensive research. A crucial factor contributing to brain aging is the alteration in microglia, the resident immune cells of the central nervous system (CNS) (Refs). Research has suggested that changes in microglial function are not just a consequence but a driver of brain aging and associated neurodegenerative diseases. This literature review aims to present a comprehensive overview of current findings related to the role of microglia in brain aging.

**An overview of microglial cells:** Microglial cells, one of the primary forms of immune defense in the CNS, have emerged as a key player in maintaining neuronal health and function (Ref). Due to aging or pathological states, a dysfunctional microglial response can contribute to neurodegeneration (Ref).

**Role of microglia in brain aging:** With aging, microglia undergo senescence-associated changes, which include alterations in morphology, function, and gene expression profiles (Ref). Aging microglia are characteristically 'primed' and exhibit a heightened response to immune stimuli, leading to increased production of pro-inflammatory cytokines (Ref).

This chronic low-grade inflammation, or 'inflammaging', may contribute to neurodegeneration and cognitive decline (Ref).

**Microglia and age-related neurodegenerative diseases:** Microglial dysfunction is linked with the progression of age-related neurodegenerative diseases like Alzheimer's disease (AD), Parkinson's disease (PD), and others (Refs). For instance, in AD, microglia fail to phagocytose efficiently and clear β-amyloid plaques, leading to their accumulation and subsequent neuronal damage (Ref).

**Challenges and future directions:** Despite ample evidence linking microglial dysregulation with brain aging, several questions remain unanswered. Some of the aspects warranting further research are the exact triggers of microglial aging, their role in the onset versus progression of neurodegenerative diseases, and whether these changes are reversible. Future studies should focus on delineating these mechanisms and exploring potential therapeutic strategies targeting microglia.

**Conclusion:** The intricate role of microglia in brain aging underlines the necessity for a comprehensive understanding of their regulatory mechanisms, dysfunctions, and impacts. The proposed preclinical study will contribute to our knowledge of microglia's role in brain aging and may reveal novel therapeutic avenues for age-related neurodegenerative disorders.

**References** Please provide the list of references used in your literature review.

**Focused groups may discuss the following questions to improve the proposal.**

**Theoretical Questions:**

- What are the current theories regarding the role of microglia in brain aging, and how might our research build on or challenge these theories?
- Are there conflicting views or theories in the literature on the role of microglia in brain aging and neurodegenerative diseases?

**Methodological Questions:**

- What specific preclinical models should we utilize for our study? Are there any new models that could offer novel insights?
- What are the strengths and weaknesses of different methods for studying microglia function and behavior?
- How will we measure and quantify 'brain aging' and microglial function?

**Ethical Considerations:**

- What ethical considerations must we keep in mind while conducting this research, mainly if we are using animal models?

**Practical and Logistical Questions:**

- What are the potential challenges in our experimental design, and how can we address these?

- Do we have the necessary resources and equipment for the study? If not, what alternatives can we consider?

**Future Implications and Applications:**

- How might our research findings contribute to the development of therapeutic strategies for age-related neurodegenerative disorders?
- What further research questions or directions might arise from our study?

**Data Analysis:**

- How will we analyze the data we collect? Do we have a plan for handling and storing large amounts of data?
- What statistical tools and methods are we planning to use and why?

**Collaboration and Communication:**

- How can we foster effective collaboration within our team and with other researchers in this field?
- How will we disseminate our findings to both the scientific community and the public?

Remember, these questions are meant to prompt discussion and may not all be relevant depending on your specific context and research goals. Adjust them as needed to fit your project

## Research Gap Example 1

*"Exploring the Impact of Social Isolation on Cognitive Decline in the Elderly Population"*

**Literature Review**: The research has extensively explored the impact of social isolation on the psychological well-being of elderly individuals. Several studies have pointed out the correlation between social isolation and increased risk of depression, anxiety, and suicide in older adults. However, a significant body of research links social interaction with cognitive function in elderly individuals.

**Identified Gap**: While the link between social isolation and mental health in the elderly has been thoroughly researched, there appears to be a research gap in understanding the direct impact of social isolation on cognitive decline in this demographic.

**Justification of the Gap**: Cognitive decline profoundly impacts the quality of life of the elderly and poses a significant public health issue. Understanding the factors contributing to cognitive decline can guide interventions and preventive measures, thereby reducing the burden on healthcare systems and improving individuals' well-being.

**Presentation of the Gap**: Existing research has not thoroughly explored the role of social isolation in cognitive decline among the elderly population. Addressing this gap will enhance our understanding of preventable risk factors associated with cognitive decline and potentially contribute to effective strategies to mitigate this issue.

**Research Question**: The research aims to answer the following question: "What is the impact of social isolation on the rate of cognitive decline in the elderly population?"

**Research Methodology**: A combination of longitudinal observational studies and neuropsychological tests will be used to measure cognitive functions over time in a sample of socially isolated elderly individuals compared to those in active social environments. This approach will allow us to measure changes in cognitive function and relate them directly to the level of social interaction.

**Expected Contribution**: The expected contribution of this research is twofold. First, it will contribute to the body of knowledge regarding the factors influencing cognitive decline in the elderly, specifically the role of social isolation. Second, it may inform the development of social programs and interventions to maintain cognitive function and reduce the burden of cognitive decline in the elderly population.

### Research Gap Example 2

*"Investigating the Effect of Novel Anti-diabetic Drug X on Beta-Cell Regeneration in Animal Models of Type 2 Diabetes"*

**Literature Review:** Several studies have demonstrated the pathophysiology of Type 2 Diabetes, focusing on insulin resistance and the gradual loss of insulin-producing beta-cells in the pancreas. Many current treatments aim to increase insulin sensitivity or provide exogenous insulin but have limited effectiveness in reversing or halting beta-cell loss. Recent research indicates a potential for beta-cell regeneration, which could revolutionize treatment paradigms.

**Identify the Gap:** However, few studies have investigated the effects of novel anti-diabetic drug X on beta-cell regeneration, particularly in the context of Type 2 Diabetes. There is an unexplored potential for this drug to promote beta-cell regeneration, which could significantly improve disease outcomes.

**Justify the Gap:** The lack of research on the impact of drug X on beta-cell regeneration in Type 2 Diabetes limits our understanding of the drug's full therapeutic potential. Given the burden of Type 2 Diabetes globally and the limitations of current therapies, it's critical to explore all potential treatment avenues.

**Present the Gap:** There is a clear research gap in understanding whether drug X can promote beta-cell regeneration in Type 2 Diabetes. Filling this gap could lead to better disease management strategies and potentially reduce the global disease burden.

**Research Question:** The main research question of this study is: "What is the effect of drug X on beta-cell regeneration in animal models of Type 2 Diabetes?"

**Research Methodology:** We propose to conduct a preclinical study using animal models with Type 2 Diabetes. After inducing diabetes in the animals, we will administer drug X and measure beta-cell mass and function, insulin levels, and blood glucose levels, comparing them with control groups. Histological and molecular analyses will be performed to evaluate the degree of beta-cell regeneration.

**Expected Contribution:** This study will contribute to our understanding of the potential of drug X in promoting beta-cell regeneration in Type 2 Diabetes. These findings could provide a basis for future clinical trials and potentially pave the way for a new treatment paradigm.

Here are two multiple-choice questions:

(1) Which of the following steps is NOT part of presenting a research gap in a proposal?

a. Conducting a literature review to understand the current state of research.

b. Identifying areas that have not been adequately addressed in the literature.

c. Justifying the gap by explaining why it is a problem that the gap exists.

d. Randomly choosing a research methodology without considering the identified gap.

(2) What is the goal of identifying and presenting a research gap in a research proposal?

a. To demonstrate that your research project is not necessary.

b. To show that you can write a long proposal.

c. To demonstrate that your research project is necessary and will contribute to the existing body of knowledge.

d. To prove that other researchers in your field are not competent.

Correct answer (1): d. Explanation: Choosing a research methodology is an essential step in the research process. However, it should be based on the research gap identified, the nature of the research problem, and the data required to answer the research question or hypothesis. Selecting a methodology randomly without considering these factors would not lead to meaningful or valid research outcomes.

Correct answer (2): c. Explanation: The goal of identifying a research gap is to showcase that your proposed research is essential and will contribute valuable new knowledge, insights, or data to the existing body of research. This helps to establish the relevance and importance of your work and can assist in securing approval or funding for your research proposal. It is not about discrediting other researchers (option d) or showing writing skills (option b), and certainly, the aim is not to prove the research unnecessary (option a).

**Hypothesis, Aim, and Objective Example 1:**

*"Dietary Fiber for Weight Management: A Randomized Controlled Trial"*

**Hypothesis:** Consuming a high-fiber diet will lead to greater weight loss and improved weight management in overweight individuals compared to a standard low-fiber diet.

**Aim:** The aim of this study is to investigate the effects of a high-fiber diet on weight management in overweight individuals through a randomized controlled trial.

**Objectives:**

1. To assess the baseline weight, body mass index (BMI), and other relevant measurements of all participants at the beginning of the study.
2. To randomly assign participants into two groups: one group will follow a high-fiber diet, and the other group will follow a low-fiber diet (control group).
3. To monitor and record the daily dietary intake of fiber for both groups during the intervention period.
4. To measure and compare the changes in weight, BMI, and waist circumference between the two groups after the intervention (e.g., after 12 weeks).
5. To analyze and compare any changes in appetite, satiety, and other relevant factors related to weight management between the high-fiber and low-fiber diet groups.
6. To assess and record any potential side effects or adverse events related to the high-fiber diet.

7. To draw conclusions based on the findings and determine whether a high-fiber diet can be an effective strategy for weight management in overweight individuals.

In an actual research proposal, you would provide the study design, sample size, data analysis methods, and ethical considerations.

**Hypothesis, Aim, and Objective Example 2:**

*"Dietary Fiber for Weight Management: A Cross-Sectional Study."*

**Hypothesis:** Individuals with higher dietary fiber intake will have lower body weight and reduced BMI than those with lower dietary fiber intake.

**Aim:** This cross-sectional study investigates the association between dietary fiber intake and weight management in a specific population.

**Objectives:**

1. To assess the dietary fiber intake of the selected population using food frequency questionnaires.
2. To measure the participant's body weight and calculate BMI (Body Mass Index).
3. To analyze the correlation between dietary fiber intake and body weight/BMI.
4. To identify any potential confounding variables (such as age, gender, physical activity levels) that might influence the relationship between dietary fiber intake and weight management.
5. To compare the differences in dietary fiber intake and weight-related variables (body weight and BMI) between different subgroups within the population (e.g., age groups, gender, etc.).
6. To discuss the implications of the findings and suggest recommendations for incorporating dietary fiber in weight management programs.

Please note that this is a simplified example, and in a complete research proposal, you would provide more in-depth information on the study's background, methodology, data analysis techniques, and limitations. Additionally, you would define the specific population you are studying and provide ethical considerations for the research

## Hypothesis, Aim, and Objective Example 3:

***Title:*** *"Polyunsaturated fatty acids n-3 in the prevention of high-fat diet-induced obesity in C57BL mice"*

**Hypothesis:** Supplementation with polyunsaturated fatty acids n-3 will *mitigate* high-fat diet-induced obesity in C57BL mice by reducing adiposity and improving metabolic markers." Explanation: The hypothesis proposes that supplementing the diet of C57BL mice with polyunsaturated fatty acids n-3 will have a preventive effect on obesity induced by a high-fat diet. It predicts that this intervention will lead to reduced adipose tissue accumulation and improved metabolic indicators.

**Aim:** This study aims to investigate the potential preventive effects of polyunsaturated fatty acids n-3 on high-fat diet-induced obesity in C57BL mice. Explanation: The aim states the overall purpose of the research, which is to examine whether polyunsaturated fatty acids n-3 can prevent obesity in C57BL mice when fed a high-fat diet. It sets the direction for the study and identifies the central question to be addressed.

**Objective Example 1:** To determine the impact of polyunsaturated fatty acids n-3 supplementation on body weight gain in C57BL mice subjected to a high-fat diet.

**Objective Example 2:** To assess the influence of polyunsaturated fatty acids n-3 supplementation on adipose tissue accumulation and distribution in C57BL mice fed a high-fat diet.

**Objective Example 3:** To examine the effects of polyunsaturated fatty acids n-3 supplementation on metabolic markers, such as glucose tolerance and insulin sensitivity, in C57BL mice on a high-fat diet.

Explanation: The objectives outline the specific goals that will be pursued to achieve the research aim. Objective 1 focuses on weight gain, Objective 2 on adipose tissue characteristics, and Objective 3 on metabolic markers. These objectives help direct the study and determine the data that needs to be collected and analyzed.

**Multiple choice questions**

1. What is a hypothesis in a research study?

   A) A broad statement of the study's purpose

   B) Specific, measurable goals derived from the research question

   C) A proposed explanation for an observed phenomenon

   D) Specific steps to accomplish the research aim

   Answer: C)

2. What does the aim of a research study represent?

   A) Specific, measurable goals derived from the research question

   B) A proposed explanation for an observed phenomenon

   C) A broad statement of the study's purpose

   D) Specific steps to accomplish the research aim

   Answer: C)

3. Which of the following best describes research objectives?

   A) Specific steps to accomplish the research aim

   B) A proposed explanation for an observed phenomenon

   C) Specific, measurable goals derived from the research question

   D) A broad statement of the study's purpose

   Answer: A)

4. What is the primary purpose of a hypothesis in a research study?

   A) To provide a broad statement of the research study's purpose

   B) To break down the overall aim into smaller, manageable steps

   C) To guide the research and testing process with a specific prediction

   D) To contextualize the research question and set the tone for the study

   Answer: C)

5. What role does the aim of a research study play?

   A) It provides specific steps to accomplish the research objectives

   B) It serves as a roadmap for the research process

C) It outlines a broad explanation for an observed phenomenon

D) It gives a high-level overview of the study's purpose

Answer: D)

6. How are research objectives related to the research question?

   A) Objectives provide a high-level overview of the research question

   B) Objectives are derived from the hypothesis to guide the study's direction

   C) Objectives break down the overall aim into specific, measurable goals

   D) Objectives serve as a roadmap for the research process

   Answer: C)

**Method Example 1**

*"Effectiveness of Mediterranean Diet in the Prevention of Type 2 Diabetes Among Prediabetic Individuals: A Randomized Controlled Trial"*

**Research Design:** This study will employ a randomized controlled trial (RCT) to examine the effectiveness of the Mediterranean diet in preventing the onset of type 2 diabetes among prediabetic individuals.

**Participants:** A total of 500 prediabetic adults aged between 30 to 60 years will be recruited for this study from health clinics within a particular region. Participants will be randomly assigned to the experimental group (n=250), who will follow the Mediterranean diet, and the control group (n=250), who will follow their regular diet. Inclusion criteria for the study include adults diagnosed as prediabetic, aged between 30 and 60, and not on a special diet due to other medical conditions.

**Data Collection Procedures:** Demographics, baseline anthropometrics, and dietary habits will be collected at the onset of the study. Follow-ups will be performed every three months over a period of two years, where anthropometrics will be measured, and dietary adherence will be assessed through 24-hour dietary recalls. Blood tests will be performed at baseline, one year, and at the end of the study to measure glucose levels and determine diabetes onset.

**Instruments:** Anthropometric measurements will be taken using a stadiometer and a calibrated scale. Dietary adherence will be assessed using a validated food frequency questionnaire. Blood tests will be conducted in a CAP-accredited laboratory.

**Data Analysis:** Data will be analyzed using an intention-to-treat approach. Continuous variables will be presented as mean ± standard deviation and categorical variables as frequencies and percentages. Time to diabetes onset will be evaluated using the Kaplan-Meier method and compared by log-rank test. Cox regression analysis will be performed to evaluate the risk of developing diabetes, adjusting for confounders. A p-value $<0.05$ will be considered statistically significant.

**Ethical Considerations:** All participants will provide written informed consent before entering the study. The research proposal has been submitted for review to the local ethical committee.

**Validity and Reliability:** The randomized controlled trial design will help ensure the study's internal validity while including a diverse range of participants from multiple clinics should enhance external validity. All measures will be taken by trained personnel to ensure data reliability.

**Limitations:** Possible limitations include the self-reported nature of dietary adherence and potential differences in physical activity levels between participants, which we will attempt to account for via questionnaires.

**Timeframe:** Recruitment and baseline data collection will take place over the first six months, with the intervention and follow-up occurring over the following two years. Data analysis and report writing are anticipated to require an additional six months.

This is just an example and might not be perfect for every situation. Always tailor the structure and content of your

Methods section to the specific requirements of your research project.

Here are some *focus group questions* that can stimulate discussion among students about the research methods used in the proposed study "Effectiveness of Mediterranean Diet in the Prevention of Type 2 Diabetes Among Prediabetic Individuals: A Randomized Controlled Trial."

1. **Understanding the Research Design**: How does the randomized controlled trial (RCT) design contribute to the validity of this study's results? Are there any other research designs that you think might be suitable for this kind of research?
2. **Data Collection Techniques**: What are the pros and cons of the data collection methods employed in this study, such as anthropometrics, dietary recalls, and blood tests? How would you ensure data accuracy and consistency?
3. **Research Instruments**: What is the importance of using a validated food frequency questionnaire in this study? How would you handle potential inaccuracies or inconsistencies in participant responses?
4. **Ethical Considerations**: What ethical issues might arise in this study, and how has the research proposal addressed them? Is there anything else you would add to the ethical considerations?
5. **Data Analysis**: Why is an intention-to-treat analysis appropriate for this study? What other statistical tests could potentially be useful, and why?

6. **Limitations**: The study acknowledges limitations such as self-reported dietary adherence and potential differences in physical activity levels between participants. How might these impact the results, and how would you propose to handle them?
7. **General Methodological Approach**: Would you have designed the study differently, given the same research question and objectives? If so, how and why?

These questions aim to encourage discussion and critical thinking about the research methods. This can deepen understanding of the principles of research design, ethical considerations, data collection, and analysis.

**Here are some potential ways to approach answering these questions:**

1. **Understanding the Research Design**: The RCT design is essential for this study because it can help establish a causal relationship between the Mediterranean diet and the prevention of type 2 diabetes. Other research designs, such as cohort or case-control studies, might provide insights but wouldn't be as definitive in proving cause-effect relationships.
2. **Data Collection Techniques**: Anthropometrics, dietary recalls, and blood tests are good data collection methods for this study because they provide objective and detailed information. However, there could be potential bias in self-reported dietary recalls, which could be minimized by thorough participant training and possibly using other dietary assessment tools like food diaries.

3. **Research Instruments**: A validated food frequency questionnaire is important because it ensures the tool has been tested for its ability to provide accurate and consistent results. Any potential inaccuracies or inconsistencies could be addressed by having a standardized questionnaire administration protocol and ensuring it's conducted by trained personnel.

4. **Ethical Considerations**: Ethical issues might include ensuring informed consent, participant privacy, and the safe handling of blood samples. The research proposal seems to address these adequately, but additional considerations might include providing dietary counseling for control group participants at the end of the study as a form of benefit sharing.

5. **Data Analysis**: An intention-to-treat analysis is appropriate for this study because it includes all participants as originally allocated after randomization. This approach helps maintain the balance of participant characteristics achieved by randomization and allows for a more real-world analysis of the intervention's effect. Other statistical tests might include a per-protocol analysis to provide additional insights.

6. **Limitations**: Self-reported dietary adherence and differences in physical activity levels could introduce bias. The study might control these factors by also tracking physical activity levels through wearable devices and considering this in the analysis, as well as having periodic checks for diet adherence.

7. **General Methodological Approach**: A student might consider supplementing the RCT design with qualitative

methods (like in-depth interviews) to gain more nuanced insights into participants' experiences with the diet, which could inform future intervention strategies.

These are general suggestions, and students can certainly delve deeper or offer alternative perspectives based on their understanding and critical thinking skills.

## Method: Example 2

*"Investigating the Role of Aerobic Exercise in Enhancing Cognitive Health in Aging: a Randomized Controlled Trial."*

**Research Design:** This study will employ a randomized controlled trial (RCT) design, which is ideal for determining causal relationships. Participants will be randomly assigned to either aerobic or control exercise groups.

**Participants:** We will recruit 200 community-dwelling adults aged 60 and above with no history of neurological disorders or other health conditions that would contraindicate aerobic exercise. Participants will be recruited through community centers and advertisements in local newspapers and online platforms. Informed consent will be obtained from all participants.

**Randomization:** Participants will be randomly assigned to either the exercise or control groups. Randomization will be conducted using computer-generated random numbers.

**Interventions:** The exercise group will participate thrice a week in a structured aerobic exercise program for 12 months. Each session will last approximately 60 minutes and will be led by a certified fitness instructor. The control group will receive standard health advice and will be asked to maintain their usual physical activity levels.

**Data Collection Procedures:** Baseline assessments will be conducted before the start of the intervention. Follow-up assessments will be carried out immediately after the intervention and six months post-intervention. Assessments will include cognitive tests, physical health measures, and lifestyle and quality of life questionnaires.

**Instruments:** Cognitive function will be assessed using the Montreal Cognitive Assessment (MoCA) and the Cambridge Neuropsychological Test Automated Battery (CANTAB). Physical fitness will be evaluated using the 6-minute walk and sit-to-stand tests.

**Data Analysis:** Data will be analyzed using SPSS software. The primary outcome will be changes in cognitive test scores. Comparisons between the exercise and control groups will be made using independent t-tests or Mann-Whitney U tests, depending on the data distribution. Changes over time within groups will be analyzed using repeated measures ANOVA or Friedman's test, as appropriate.

**Ethical Considerations:** All procedures will follow the institutional research committee's ethical standards, the 1964 Helsinki Declaration, and its later amendments or comparable ethical standards.

**Validity and Reliability:** The RCT design, the use of validated instruments, and the plan to conduct intention-to-treat analysis will contribute to the validity and reliability of the study.

**Limitations:** Potential limitations include the risk of dropouts, which may introduce bias, and the reliance on self-report for lifestyle variables, which may be subject to recall bias.

**Timeframe:** The study is expected to take approximately 18 months to complete, including three months for recruitment, 12 months for the intervention, and three months for data analysis and report writing.

Actual research proposals would likely include more detail on each of these points and potentially additional sub-sections, depending on the nature of the study and the requirements of the funding body or ethical review board.

Here are some multiple-choice questions.

(1) What type of research design will be used in the proposed study?

a. Observational

b. Cross-sectional

c. Cohort

d. Randomized controlled trial

Answer: d.

(2) How will participants be assigned to the exercise or control group?

a. Based on their current fitness level

b. Based on their age

c. Randomly, using computer-generated random numbers

d. Based on their cognitive test scores

Answer: c.

(3) What primary instruments are used to assess cognitive function?

a. The Hamilton Depression Scale and Beck Anxiety Inventory

b. The Stanford-Binet Intelligence Scale and Wechsler Adult Intelligence Scale

c. The Montreal Cognitive Assessment (MoCA) and Cambridge Neuropsychological Test Automated Battery (CANTAB)

d. The Trail Making Test and Stroop Test

Answer: c.

(4) What potential limitation is acknowledged in the research proposal?

a. The cost of hiring a fitness instructor for the exercise group

b. The difficulty of obtaining computer-generated random numbers

c. The risk of dropouts and reliance on self-report for lifestyle variables

d. The inability to use SPSS software for data analysis

Answer: c.

## Method Example 3:

*Clozapine affects microglia: A possible mechanism through brain immunity?*

This proposal aims to investigate the underlying mechanisms that potentially make clozapine a more effective antipsychotic treatment option for patients who have proven to be resistant to other forms of antipsychotic drug treatments, with a focus on the potential role of brain immunity. This study will utilize both in vitro and in vivo models.

### 1. Research Design

This will be an experimental study incorporating both qualitative and quantitative research methods. The primary focus will be exploring the effect of clozapine on human microglial cells *in vitro* and *in vivo* through the use of the Caenorhabditis elegans (C. elegans) model.

### 2. Experimental Models

*In Vitro Model*

We will use an established human microglia cell line for the in vitro component of the study. These cells will be cultured and maintained in a controlled environment following standard protocols. The cells will be divided into two groups: a control group (treated with a vehicle) and an experimental group (treated with various concentrations of clozapine).

*In Vivo Model*

The C. elegans model will be used for the in vivo part of the study. C. elegans is a well-established model organism for neurobiological research due to its simple nervous system and conserved neural genes. We will use a wild-type control and a transgenic strain expressing human immune response-related genes. These worms will be exposed to control or clozapine-enriched environments.

**3. Data Collection**

The effect of clozapine on human microglia cells will be assessed through cell viability assays, inflammation-related gene and protein expression assays, and morphological analysis.

In the C. elegans model, we will investigate the effects of clozapine exposure on behavior (using established behavioral assays such as locomotion and feeding), survival, and immune response gene expression.

**4. Data Analysis**

Data analysis will be performed using statistical software. The Student's t-test or ANOVA will be used to compare the means of two or more independent groups, while the Chi-squared test or Fisher's exact test will be employed for categorical data.

*In vitro* experiments will evaluate gene and protein expression changes and cell viability between control and clozapine-treated microglia. This will allow for the identification of potential molecular pathways activated by clozapine.

In the C. elegans model, the effects of clozapine on survival, behavior, and immune response gene expression will be analyzed. Survival curves will be generated using the Kaplan-Meier method and compared using the Log-rank (Mantel-Cox) test.

The Spearman's or Pearson's correlation coefficients will be computed to determine the relationships between different parameters in the study. A p-value of less than 0.05 will be considered statistically significant.

**5. Validity and Reliability:** To ensure the validity and reliability of the study, we will perform all experiments in triplicate and repeat at least three times independently. Also, all experimental procedures will be carried out blind to reduce bias.

**6. Ethical Considerations:** Although our study does not directly involve human participants, we will still uphold all ethical guidelines related to the use of human cell lines and animal models. The study involving C. elegans will follow the guidelines the local animal care and use committee set out.

In conclusion, these methods are intended to shed light on how clozapine might mediate its unique efficacy in treatment-resistant patients, potentially illuminating new pathways for future therapeutic strategies.

## Focused Group Discussion 1: Improving *In Vitro* and *In Vivo* Models

The discussion will revolve around the best practices to enhance the results of the in vitro and in vivo studies. Some possible topics could include:

1. What specific markers of inflammation and immune response should we focus on in the human microglial cell line study?
2. Can we implement additional cell lines to validate our findings?

3. Can we consider the short vs. long-term application of clozapine to understand drug efficacy in real-world settings?

Focused Group Discussion 2: Enhancing Data Collection and Analysis

This discussion aims to improve the data collection and analysis procedures. This could encompass:

1. Are there more efficient ways to measure gene and protein expression?
2. Are there more comprehensive ways to capture behavioral changes in C. elegans beyond locomotion and feeding?
3. Should we consider a multi-variate analysis approach given the likely multifactorial nature of clozapine's effects?
4. Can we implement machine learning or other advanced statistical methods to find patterns in our data?

A summarized comparison between research design and experiment design

| **Aspect** | **Research Design** | **Experiment Design** |
|---|---|---|
| **Scope** | Overall plan for a research study. | Specific plan for an experiment within research. |
| **Components** | Objectives, hypotheses, data types, collection methods, analyses. | Selection of subjects, random assignment, control of variables, manipulation of independent variable. |
| **Types** | Descriptive, Correlational, Experimental, Quasi-experimental, Exploratory, Cross-sectional, Longitudinal. | True Experimental, Factorial, Repeated Measures, Matched Pairs. |
| **Purpose** | Guides entire research process for valid results. | Establish cause-and-effect relationship through controlled conditions. |

**Research Design Example 1:**

Title: The Impact of Dietary Fiber Intake on Body Weight Management in Adults

1. Objective: To determine whether increased dietary fiber intake correlates with body weight management in adults.
2. Hypotheses:
    - Adults consuming higher amounts of dietary fiber have lower body weights than those consuming lesser amounts.
    - Higher fiber intake is associated with decreased caloric intake.
3. Data Type: Quantitative – measurements of dietary fiber intake (grams/day), body weight (kg), and daily caloric intake (kcal/day).
4. Data Collection Methods:
    - Dietary Assessment: 7-day food diary to quantify daily fiber intake.
    - Weight Measurement: Standardized weight scales.
    - Caloric Intake: Analysis of the food diary.
5. Analyses:
    - Correlation between fiber intake and body weight.
    - Correlation between fiber intake and caloric intake.

**Experimental Design Example 2:**

Title: The Effect of Increased Fiber Intake on Body Weight Over a 12-Week Period

1. Subjects: 60 adults, aged 25-45 years, with a BMI between 25 and 30 (overweight range).
2. Random Assignment:
    - Control Group (n=30): No change in diet.
    - Experimental Group (n=30): Introduction of a daily fiber supplement (e.g., psyllium husk) in addition to their regular diet.
3. Manipulated Variable: The introduction of the daily fiber supplement.
4. Controlled Variables:
    - Activity levels (e.g., ensure all participants engage in similar physical activity).
    - Total caloric intake (e.g., maintain a consistent daily intake across both groups).
    - Other dietary components (e.g., protein, fat, and carbohydrate intake).
5. Measurements:
    - Weekly body weight.
    - Weekly analysis of food diaries for consistency and adherence.
6. Outcome:
    - Change in body weight after the 12-week period.

## Expected Outcome Example 1:

"Effectiveness of Mediterranean Diet in the Prevention of Type 2 Diabetes Among Prediabetic Individuals: A Randomized Controlled Trial".

1. **Improved Glucose Tolerance**: We anticipate that the adoption of a Mediterranean diet will improve glucose tolerance in prediabetic individuals, as evidenced by a decrease in HbA1c levels.
2. **Weight Management**: We expect that the prediabetic individuals who adhere to the Mediterranean diet will maintain or achieve a healthier weight, reducing obesity-related risks associated with the progression to Type 2 diabetes.
3. **Reduction in the Progression to Type 2 Diabetes**: Our primary expected outcome is a statistically significant reduction in the progression from prediabetes to type 2 diabetes in the group following the Mediterranean diet compared to the control group.
4. **Improved Cardiovascular Health**: Given that the Mediterranean diet is rich in heart-healthy fats, we anticipate an improvement in cardiovascular health markers such as reduced LDL cholesterol and triglycerides levels, and increased HDL cholesterol levels.
5. **Evidence for Diet Recommendations**: By demonstrating the effectiveness of a Mediterranean diet in preventing the progression to type 2 diabetes, this research could provide evidence-based dietary recommendations for prediabetic individuals and high-risk populations.

6. **Increased Quality of Life**: We anticipate that adhering to the Mediterranean diet may improve participants' quality of life due to factors like weight loss and the general health benefits associated with the Mediterranean dietary pattern. This outcome will be assessed using validated quality-of-life questionnaires.
7. **Expanded Understanding of Disease Prevention**: Lastly, this research will contribute to the broader understanding of the role of diet in the prevention of chronic diseases like type 2 diabetes.

These outcomes should be measured through relevant metrics to support the results. For example, blood tests to monitor glucose levels, lipid profile, HbA1c levels, weight tracking, or validated surveys for quality of life

Here are some examples of how you might write expected outcomes for a research proposal investigating the effects of a new diabetes medication:

- We anticipate the new drug will reduce fasting blood sugar levels by 10-20% in 75% of trial participants after six months of treatment.
- We expect participants to experience fewer side effects than the current leading diabetes medication, improving adherence to the treatment regimen.
- We project a significant decrease in HbA1c levels, indicating better long-term blood glucose control.

- Through this research, we expect to contribute to current diabetes treatment practices by providing a more effective and better-tolerated treatment option.

Remember to be realistic in your expected outcomes - don't overpromise what your research can deliver. As your research progresses, you might need to refine these expected outcomes based on your actual findings.

## Validity: Example 1

*The Effects of Increased Dietary Fiber Intake on Type 2 Diabetes Management*

A research proposal examining the effects of dietary fiber on health, with a specific focus on addressing validity:

**Methodology:** "Our research will utilize a longitudinal, observational study design to investigate the long-term effects of increased dietary fiber intake on glycemic control in patients with type 2 diabetes.

**Internal Validity:** To increase internal validity, we will control for confounding variables such as age, sex, physical activity levels, and other dietary factors that could influence blood glucose levels. Furthermore, our data analysis will use multivariable regression analysis to account for these potential confounders.

**External Validity:** To enhance external validity, the project will recruit a diverse group of participants in terms of age, gender, ethnicity, and socio-economic status. This broad participant base will allow for a wider generalization of our findings.

**Construct Validity:** For construct validity, 'glycemic control' will be determined by measuring hemoglobin A1c (HbA1c) levels, a reliable and standard clinical measure for long-term glucose management. 'Dietary fiber intake' will be quantified using a validated food frequency questionnaire alongside 24-hour dietary recalls.

**Content Validity:** To ensure content validity, we will not limit our study to a specific type of dietary fiber (soluble or insoluble) but examine the overall fiber intake from all dietary sources.

**Criterion-related Validity:** To establish criterion-related validity, we will correlate the amount of dietary fiber intake with changes in HbA1c levels over time.

Potential limitations that may affect the validity of our findings include inaccurate self-reporting of dietary intake and non-adherence to dietary recommendations. To mitigate these, we will provide clear instructions for recording dietary intake and conduct regular follow-ups to encourage adherence."

In this way, we're accounting for the study's validity in the design, methodology, and analysis. Addressing validity in your research proposal is crucial, as it indicates that you have considered and planned for potential sources of bias or error in your study.

Here are two multiple-choice questions based on the example of the research proposal about the effects of increased dietary fiber intake on type 2 diabetes management:

(1) Which method will be used to improve internal validity in this study?

A. Participants will be assigned to a control group or a treatment group.

B. The study will recruit a diverse group of participants in terms of age, gender, ethnicity, and socio-economic status.

C. The design should control for confounding variables such as age, sex, physical activity levels, and other dietary factors.

D. The study will focus on overall fiber intake from all dietary sources.

Answer: C. Confounding variables such as age, sex, physical activity levels, and other dietary factors will be controlled for.

(2) How will construct validity be ensured in this study?

A. By using a longitudinal, observational study design.

B. By using multivariable regression analysis to account for potential confounders in the data analysis.

C. 'Glycemic control' will be determined by measuring hemoglobin A1c (HbA1c) levels and 'dietary fiber intake' will be quantified using a validated food frequency questionnaire.

D. By correlating the amount of dietary fiber intake with changes in HbA1c levels over time.

Answer: C. 'Glycemic control' will be determined by measuring hemoglobin A1c (HbA1c) levels, and 'dietary fiber intake' will be quantified using a validated food frequency questionnaire.

### Validity Example 2

*The Impact of Regular Aerobic Exercise on Glycemic Control in Individuals with Type 2 Diabetes*

A research proposal examining the effects of aerobic exercise on type 2 diabetes management, with emphasis on addressing validity:

**Methodology:** "Our research will implement a randomized controlled trial (RCT) to investigate the effects of regular aerobic exercise on glycemic control in individuals with type 2 diabetes.

**Internal Validity:** To ensure internal validity, we will randomly assign participants to either an intervention group, which will follow a specific aerobic exercise regimen, or a control group, which will maintain their usual physical activity levels. All participants will continue with their standard diabetes treatment plan to control the effects of medication on blood glucose levels.

**External Validity:** To promote external validity and the generalizability of our results, we will recruit a diverse sample of individuals with type 2 diabetes, covering a range of ages, ethnicities, and both genders.

**Construct Validity:** For construct validity, we will measure glycemic control using HbA1c levels, a standard and reliable measure of long-term blood glucose control. The exercise regimen will be quantified using exercise logs and wearable activity trackers to accurately capture the frequency, duration, and intensity of participants' aerobic exercise.

**Content Validity:** Our intervention, aerobic exercise, will not be limited to one specific activity (e.g., running). Participants in the intervention group will be advised to engage in any form of aerobic exercise (e.g., swimming, cycling, brisk walking) to ensure content validity.

**Criterion-related Validity:** Criterion-related validity will be established by correlating the extent of participation in aerobic exercise (as indicated by the exercise logs and activity trackers) with changes in HbA1c levels over the study period.

We anticipate potential limitations such as individual variations in adherence to the exercise program and variations in diet which might influence blood glucose levels. We will address these by providing regular follow-ups and motivational support to encourage adherence, and we will monitor dietary intake using food diaries to account for dietary influences in our analysis."

This example demonstrates how to address validity in a research proposal using an intervention-based study design. The approach might vary based on the nature of the research and the methods used, but the principles of ensuring and addressing validity remain the same.

Here are two multiple-choice questions based on the above example.

(1) In the proposed study on the impact of regular aerobic exercise on glycemic control in individuals with type 2 diabetes, which of the following methods will be used to ensure internal validity?

a) Participants will be assigned randomly to the intervention or control group.

b) The sample will include diverse ages, ethnicities, and genders.

c) Participants will be advised to engage in aerobic exercise.

d) Glycemic control will be measured using HbA1c levels.

(2) How will the researchers quantify the intervention to establish construct validity in the same study?

a) By measuring HbA1c levels.

b) By providing regular follow-ups and motivational support.

c) By using food diaries to monitor dietary intake.

d) By using exercise logs and wearable activity trackers.

Here are the correct answers to the questions:

(1) The correct answer is (a) Participants will be assigned randomly to the intervention or control group. This random assignment helps ensure that any observed effects on glycemic control can be attributed to the intervention (regular aerobic exercise), rather than other factors, which increases internal validity.

**(2)** The correct answer is (d). By using exercise logs and wearable activity trackers. These tools will be used to accurately capture the frequency, duration, and intensity of participants' aerobic exercise, thereby providing a quantifiable measure of the intervention and contributing to construct validity.

## Significance Example

Our research proposal aims to investigate the effectiveness of a new treatment approach for managing Alzheimer's disease. Despite extensive research, there remains no cure for Alzheimer's, and current treatments only manage symptoms, leaving a significant gap in care. Alzheimer's disease affects millions of people worldwide and is a leading cause of disability and dependency among older people, signifying the pressing need for better treatment options.

Our research proposes a novel therapeutic strategy based on recent molecular biology discoveries, demonstrating our study's innovative nature. If successful, our research could lead to more effective treatments that manage symptoms and potentially slow disease progression. This could dramatically improve the quality of life for Alzheimer's patients and their caregivers.

Moreover, more effective treatments could reduce the economic burden of Alzheimer's disease, which costs billions of dollars each year in healthcare expenses and lost productivity. By pioneering a new approach, our study could open avenues for further research, contributing to the long-term goal of finding a cure for Alzheimer's disease."

CHAPTER 2

# Effective Literature Search

**TOPIC OUTLINE**

Overview
Guidelines

## Overview

A *literature search* is essential before starting to plan a research project. It helps in understanding the research topic and developing a research question.

Today, the available data in the literature is massive; thus, selecting the relevant and appropriate papers is extremely important. Knowing how to search for the documents can help the research design, save time, and ensure you focus on critical issues.

Conducting an effective literature search is an essential step in any research project. It ensures that you understand the existing body of knowledge on your topic, which allows you to build upon it, find gaps in current understanding, and avoid replicating previous studies.

## Guidelines

*Research question:* The first step is to develop a research question in a research area. The well-known approaches to forming a research question are (1) to contain patients, intervention, comparison, outcome, and time (PICOT) and (2) to be feasible, interesting, novel, ethical, and relevant (FINER). Start with a broad topic. Narrow it down to a specific question or set of questions.

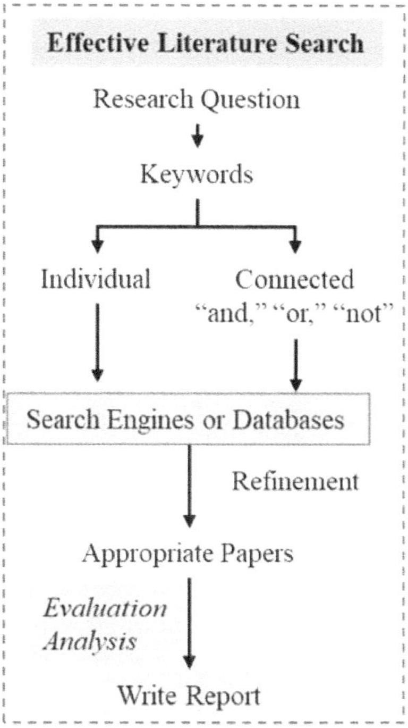


Identify Keywords and Phrases: Break down your research question into its core concepts. Think of synonyms, related terms, and alternate spellings for each concept.

*Search engines:* Google and Google Scholar are search engines frequently used in biomedical paper searches.

*Choose Relevant Databases and Platforms: 1)* Academic Databases: PubMed (for life sciences), Web of Science, Scopus, Google Scholar, and specialized databases related to your field. 2) University Libraries: Access to subscriptions and additional resources. 3) Other Resources: Books, theses, reports, conference proceedings, etc

*Literature types:* (1) peer-reviewed articles and conference papers, (2) systematic review and meta-analysis, (3) reference books.

*Words used for searching:* Write down your main ideas, synonyms, related words, and phrases.

*Connect the search words:* Find results with one or more search words:

- *And:* Find papers that mention both words. You may search for an idea using "and" between the keywords. *Example:* "obesity and a high-fat diet." This will find papers with both of the search words.
- *Or:* Widen the search using "or" between words. This will find more articles than searching one word. This is because "or" means the same thing. Example: "obesity or body mass index." This search will find articles with either or both of the search words.
- *Not:* Narrowing the search using "not" between words. This will search papers containing the first word but not the second. Example: "aged population, not young adult."

*Truncation (*):* The asterisk symbol (*) will help you search for different word endings. *Example:* "Cover*" will find results with the words *cover, coverage, covers.*

*Phrase searching "……":* Double quotation marks help you search for a common phrase and make your results more relevant. *Example:* "cognitive impairment" will find results with the words *cognitive impairment* together as a phrase.

*Refinement:* Focusing on the topic, you can narrow and refine your search results using the following strategies.

- Year of publication or date range (for recent or historical research)
- Document or source type, e.g., randomized controlled trial, review, survey, or book

*Research types:* If you're looking for particular types of research, you can use these as search words. *Example:* qualitative, quantitative, and methodology.

*Evaluation:*

- A paper evaluation includes identifying (1) the main point relevant to your research project, (2) the quality of the data (e.g., sample size, appropriate techniques used), and (3) pitfalls.

*Synthesize data and analysis:*

- Having all the relevant papers, you may start synthesizing the data and conducting the investigation. Then, finally, you can produce a report.

*Review the Literature:*

- Skim the abstracts to decide which articles to read in full.
- Note the methodologies, results, and conclusions of each study.

- Identify patterns, trends, gaps, or controversies in the literature.

# Example

You may be interested in doing a research project on "Long-term effects of Mediterranean diet on cognitive function in elderly individuals." Conducting an effective literature search is a crucial step in the research process. Here's a step-by-step guide to help you get started:

**1. Define your research question:** Clearly articulate your research question or objective. In your case, it's about the long-term effects of the Mediterranean diet on cognitive function in elderly individuals.

**2. Identify keywords and synonyms:** List keywords and synonyms related to your research topic. These could include terms like "Mediterranean diet," "cognitive function," "elderly," "long-term effects," and related concepts.

**3. Choose appropriate databases:** Select relevant academic databases to search for scholarly articles. Common health and nutrition research databases include PubMed, Web of Science, Google Scholar, and PsycINFO.

**4. Start with a broad search:** Begin with a broad search using your chosen keywords. This will give you an overview of the existing literature on your topic.

**5. Review search results**: Browse through the search results and read the titles and abstracts to identify potentially relevant articles. Pay attention to the study design, population, and key findings.

**6. Refine your search:** As you review the initial results, you'll likely identify more specific terms or concepts that are relevant. Use these insights to refine your search, making it more targeted.

**7. Use citation tracking:** If you find a key article that's highly relevant to your research, use citation tracking to see who has cited that article. This can help you discover more recent research on the same topic.

**8. Analyze and synthesize:** As you review the articles, take notes on key findings, study methodologies, sample sizes, and other relevant details. Synthesize the information to identify common themes, trends, and gaps in the literature.

**9. Write your literature review:** Once thoroughly reviewing and analyzing the articles, use your findings to write a comprehensive literature review section for your research project.

Remember that conducting a literature search is an iterative process. You may need to refine your search terms and strategies as you go along. Also, ensure that you critically evaluate the quality and credibility of the sources you include in your research.

PART TWO

# Paper Writing

*Purpose:* Medical research has a long history back to the biblical descriptions in 500 BC; however, the primary goal has not changed. The path of medical research has moved from diets, herbs, and exercise to drugs. However, the direct purposes of medical research have never changed; they are to improve human health, find better ways to treat and prevent diseases, and understand the pathology and mechanism of the disease occurring. The medical research paper is essential in disseminating medical news, including therapy, prevention, and knowledge. In addition, medical papers are the place for the discussion and debate of opinions and idea discrepancies and different findings.

*Researchers:* Researchers should put their research outcomes in the public domain. A research paper can be either large or small, positive or negative. Publishing the research findings will help other researchers improve their work, thus contributing to the body of knowledge in the research field. In addition, the researchers need to put their work beyond their narrow topic in the relevant large research area. By publishing quality papers, researchers can build up their credentials.

*Paper types:* Medical papers can be *full* or *not full.* Full papers include research and review papers; however, not full papers are brief communications, commentaries, or perspectives. Others, including conference abstracts and commercial and contract reports, do not count as research papers.

*Paper structure:* Research papers have unique features and designs accepted worldwide, although different journals require some variations. Therefore, we do not recommend creating a new style of research paper; instead, you should follow the standard format all researchers use. Finally, you should check the paper format requirements instructed by the journal where you intend to submit your paper for publication.

The structure of a research paper is similar among all journals, although there are some variations, including title, abstract, introduction, materials and methods, results, discussions, references, and acknowledgment.

## A general template for writing a research paper

Title: Your research topic title, succinct and informative

Authors: Your name, co-authors, affiliations

Abstract:

- Brief summary of the research problem.
- Methodology employed.
- Principal results.
- Major conclusions.
- Keywords: [4-6 key terms related to your research]

1. Introduction

- Background of the study.
- Importance of the research topic.
- Purpose of the study.
- Research questions or hypotheses.
- The literature review should include: 1) Overview of the key literature in your field; 2) Identify gaps or unresolved issues in the existing literature; 3) Justify the need for your research.

3. Methodology

- Research Design: Describe the overall approach (e.g., experimental, qualitative, quantitative).
- Participants: Details about the sample population (if applicable).
- Instruments: Tools used for data collection (e.g., questionnaires, software).
- Procedure: Steps followed during the research.
- Data Analysis: Techniques used to analyze the data.

4. Results

- Present the findings using appropriate means (tables, figures).
- Use subsections if needed to break up and organize results.

5. Discussion

- Interpret the results in relation to the research questions or hypotheses.
- Compare your findings with the literature reviewed.
- Limitations of your study.
- Implications of your results.

6. Conclusion

- Summarize the main findings.
- State the significance of the study.
- Recommendations for further research or application.

Acknowledgments

- Thank anyone who supported or helped during the research process.

References

- List all sources cited in the paper in a consistent

CHAPTER 3

# Research Paper

**TOPIC OUTLINE**

Title
Abstract
Introduction
Material and methods
Research design
Results, tables, figures
Discussion
Paper submission
Science citation index
Journal impact factor
What is the h-index?

What is a research paper? A *research paper* is a complete data report after completing a research project. This type of publication is the most common among research publications. It should not be a truncated story or simple data communication. A research paper is also called an *original research paper* or a *research report.*

Types of research papers: A medical research paper can be a human-, animal-, or cell-based study, depending on the research question that the researcher wants to answer.

## Essential Criteria

*Novelty:* Novelty is essential when you publish a research paper. It contains original research, including new ideas, novel findings, or new methods that have not been previously published.

*Quality:* Quality must reach a high standard, including reliable data and convincing discoveries.

*Systematic:* A systematic approach means a complete investigation of a research question. The report should provide a full story, not truncated material, with a clear and logical text flow.

## Title

The title of a paper should include the main ideas and content of the research. It should also be exciting and use some keywords.

A preferred title is descriptive or declarative and should allow for content prediction. Keep the title concise, and avoid jargon and unnecessary words. You could also cover the method and sample size. Usually, the title is finalized at the end of paper writing.

*Why is the title important?* Readers always see the title first and read the title carefully. A good title attracts the reader's attention, is more likely to be remembered, and can lead to more citations.

### Here are some examples:

*A title emphasizes variables:* The paper title focuses on the variables and their relations. It can be an independent variable versus a dependent variable. *Example:* "A New Aerobic *Protocol* Improves Learning *Efficacy* in Adolescent Schoolchildren." It can be between two independent variables. *Example:* "Sex-Based Difference in Skeletal Muscle Fiber Type Composition in Response to Estrogen

Treatment." Here, the independent variables are male and female. The outcome variable is the muscle fiber type composition.

*A title emphasizes the conclusion:* The paper title gives an exciting conclusion to the experiment. It can be a patient outcome. *Example:* "Beneficial Effects of Walnuts on Cognition and Brain Health in Alzheimer's Disease." The title can talk about a function. *Example:* "Physical Exercise Improves Cognitive Function." "Bad Weather Induces Low Emotion on a Cold Morning in the Northern Part of India."

*A title emphasizes the effect and role:* The paper title can emphasize a positive or negative impact. *Example:* "Dietary Fiber Intake Is Positively Related to Cognitive Function" (positive) or "A Fiber-Deprived Diet Causes Cognitive Impairment" (negative). It can have two phrases. *Example:* "Obesity-Associated Inflammation: Does Curcumin Play a Beneficial Role?"

## Avoid Vagueness in a Title

*An unanswerable question:* A paper title should not use an unanswerable question. *Example:* "How Does a High-Fat Diet Cause Obesity?" This question cannot be answered. Instead, try to use the title to state the facts. *Example:* "A High-Fat Diet Promotes Weight Gain and Obesity."

*Too broad:* A paper title should avoid generic titles, which a single investigation cannot answer. *Example:* "The Role of a High-Fat Diet in Obesity."

*Abbreviations:* A paper title should avoid abbreviations, jargon, or terms. *Example:* "DIO Mice Prefer to Take HF Food Even on a Pair Feeding."

*Similarity:* Be mindful of the existing literature to avoid similar titles and concepts.

## Style the Title

*Capitalize the correct words:* We suggest capitalizing certain words in the title, including the first word, last word, and every other word except conjunctions, prepositions, and articles (though style requirements may vary). Avoid capitalizing all words or using all caps on the words in the title. (See examples above).

*Punctuation:* There is no need to have a period at the end of the title. If the title asks a question, use a question mark at the end, and if it is exclamatory, use an exclamation mark. Colons are good inside a title to break up multiple parts. *Example:* "Obesity-Associated Inflammation: Does Curcumin Play a Beneficial Role?"

## Examples

A good title should be concise, informative, and reflect your research's central theme. It should be clear, concise, and specific. It should offer readers a snapshot of the study's main focus and method without being overly wordy or vague. Here are some examples of good and bad research titles for obesity research, along with explanations:

## Good Research Titles

The Association Between Fast Food Consumption and Childhood Obesity in Urban Areas. Why is this a good title? This title is specific, focusing on fast food consumption and its link to childhood obesity in urban areas.

Metabolic and Hormonal Responses to High-Intensity Interval Training in Obese Adults. Why is this a good title? It specifies the type of exercise being studied (High-Intensity Interval Training) and the population of interest (Obese Adults). The mention of metabolic and hormonal responses provides insight into the mechanisms being studied.

The Impact of School-based Nutrition Interventions on Adolescent BMI: A Systematic Review. Why is this a good title? The title is clear about the type of intervention (school-based nutrition interventions), the target population (adolescents), and the research method (a systematic review).

**Bad Research Titles:**

“Why Are People Fat?” This title is too broad and lacks specificity. It doesn't provide clear information about the focus or methodology of the research.

“Looking at Obesity Stuff in Kids” Informal language (like "stuff") is unprofessional and vague. "Looking at" is also passive and doesn't specify what aspect of "obesity stuff" is being studied.

“Exercise and Obesity: Things to Know” While slightly more specific than the previous titles, "Things to Know" is still too vague and doesn't give a clear sense of the research's purpose or approach.

## Abstract

An abstract is a summary of the paper. It ensures readers can quickly understand the work and main ideas before reading the entire article. Sometimes, an abstract can contain findings instead of detailed results. An abstract can also report unexpected findings but omit preliminary or uncertain results. An abstract can include the method of the results, meaning how the outcome was generated, but there is no need to provide a detailed explanation.

*When do you need to write an abstract?* It is common to provide an abstract when you publish a research paper and conference report or submit a report, research proposal, or thesis proposal.

*Length:* The abstract length can usually vary from 150 to 250 words. The word count depends on the requirement of the journal or reporting body. The abstract should aim at presenting a story if it is an unstructured abstract. In this case, the method would have to be short or embedded in the results.

*Structured and unstructured abstracts:* There are two types of abstracts: structured and unstructured. Both formats should contain background, methods, results, discussion, and conclusions. In a structured abstract, the author writes the above items in separate sections. You could describe the participants, intervention protocol, technique, and measurement given a structured abstract. However, if you want to write an unstructured abstract, these items will not be separated and will be written in a single paragraph without separation.

In the end, the abstract should have a conclusion and significance. The former is to synthesize the meaning of all findings. The latter aims to point out the external validity of the findings or implications of the research.

**An example of a good abstract**

Title: The Efficacy of Intermittent Fasting in Reducing Obesity Rates: A Randomized Controlled Trial

Abstract:

Background: Obesity, a global health issue, has been linked to numerous chronic conditions. There is increasing interest in intermittent fasting (IF) as an effective weight management strategy.

Objective: To investigate the effects of intermittent fasting on body weight and metabolic markers in adults with obesity.

Methods: A 12-month randomized controlled trial included 400 participants (BMI ≥ 30 kg/m^2). Participants were assigned to either an intermittent fasting group (8-hour eating window) or a regular diet control group. Outcomes measured included body weight, BMI, fasting blood glucose, and cholesterol levels.

Results: At 12 months, the IF group experienced significant reductions in body weight (-7.2±2.1kg, $p<0.001$), BMI (-2.8±0.8, $p<0.001$), and fasting blood glucose (-5.3±1.9 mg/dL, $p<0.05$) compared to the control group.

Conclusion: Intermittent fasting offers a promising approach to weight loss and metabolic improvement in obese individuals. Further large-scale studies are warranted.

## An example of a poorly written abstract

Title: Intermittent Fasting and Weight Loss

Abstract:

Obesity is a big problem. Many people are talking about intermittent fasting (or IF) as a potential way to deal with this. We did a study on 400 people to see if it works. Some were told to do IF, and some were not. After 12 months, the ones who did IF lost more weight than those who didn't. They also had better blood test results. We think IF might be good for losing weight, but more research is needed.

The good abstract is well-structured and clearly communicates the objective, methods, results, and conclusion of the study. On the other hand, the bad abstract is informal, lacks structure, and omits crucial details about the study, making it less informative and less professional.

**Here are several multiple-choice questions based on the above abstract examples:**

Question 1: Which of the following statements best represents the objective of the study in the "Good Abstract"?

a) Obesity is a significant health problem.

b) Many people discuss intermittent fasting.

c) To investigate the effects of intermittent fasting on body weight and metabolic markers in adults with obesity.

d) The participants were observed for 12 months.

Correct Answer: c) To investigate the effects of intermittent fasting on body weight and metabolic markers in adults with obesity. Why: The "Objective" section in the good abstract clearly states the aim of the study as investigating the effects of intermittent fasting on body weight and metabolic markers in obese adults.

Question 2: At the end of 12 months, how did the weight loss in the Intermittent Fasting group compare to the control group, according to the "Good Abstract"?

a) The IF group gained more weight than the control group.

b) There was no difference in weight loss between the two groups.

c) The IF group lost significantly more weight than the control group.

d) The study did not measure weight loss.

Correct Answer: c) The IF group lost significantly more weight than the control group. Why: The "Results" section in the good abstract states that the IF group experienced significant reductions in body weight compared to the control group.

Question 3: Which of the following best describes the tone and structure of the "Bad Abstract"?

a) Professional and detailed.

b) Informal and lacks crucial study details.

c) Primarily focused on the methods used.

d) Discusses the global implications of obesity.

Correct Answer: b) Informal and lacks crucial study details. Why: The "Bad Abstract" is written in an informal tone ("Obesity is a big problem", "Many people are talking about", "We did a study"), and it doesn't provide structured details on the objective, methods, results, or conclusions as seen in the good abstract.

## Introduction

The introduction serves as a justification for the motivation and reason for the study. It informs the reader of what is going on in a particular field, the research gap, hypothesis, or aim. Therefore, the introduction should be very focused and narrow compared to the discussion.

*Research question:* The introduction should address the research story and the rationale for the research question and explain why the questions being asked are relevant. The research question should occur in the context of an already formed body of knowledge. What is the issue or problem that the study aims to address? The introduction must point out "known versus unknown." *Example:* The antipsychotic drug treats psychosis but can cause weight gain as a side effect. The mechanism facilitating this side-effect is unknown.

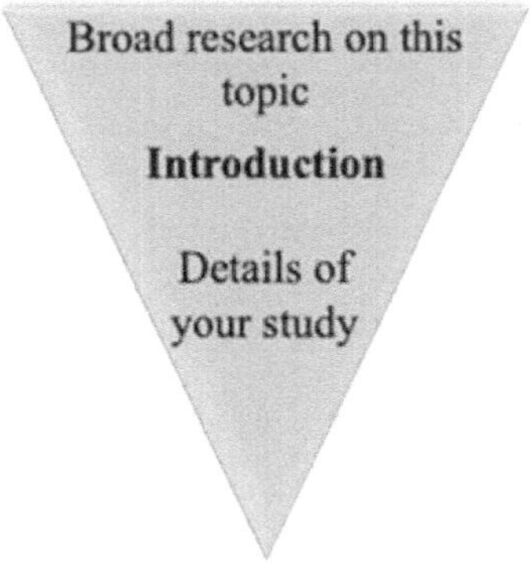


The figure above shows that the way to write the introduction is to begin with the broad research field and then gradually narrow it down to the specific questions.

## Structure of an Introduction

*Topic:* The research topic is the research area. A concise description leads readers to the point of the research. The topic should not be too broad, nor should it be too specific.

*Gap:* The research gap will be the research topic of the paper. It can be a knowledge gap, clinical problem, or something not yet known. It should have a clear focus.

*Justification:* The research justification is a connection between the topic and gap, which requires reason and specificity.

*Purpose:* The research purpose is the aim or hypothesis that this study wants to achieve or investigate.

## Checklist for the Introduction

1. Does the introduction justify the necessity of the study?
2. Does the introduction inform the reader of what is happening in the particular field?
3. Was the first sentence of interest to the reader?
4. Was there clear evidence to support the research topic?
5. As the research question is introduced, does it contain PICOT?
6. Was the hypothesis or aim clearly described at the end?
7. Were the citations current and logical?

## Styles

There are two styles of research paper introductions, each having different emphases.

*First style:* The first style emphasizes or justifies the reasons and motivations for the study. It describes what is known and unknown, why the research is required, and the study's purpose and hypothesis.

*Second style:* The second style introduces the entire paper's content or story. It covers what is known and unknown, why the research is necessary, and its main findings and conclusions.

Many high-impact journals use the second style, as the introduction section starts with the research justification, gap, and aims. Then, the researcher describes the main findings, methods, and conclusions. This presents a summary of the entire paper.

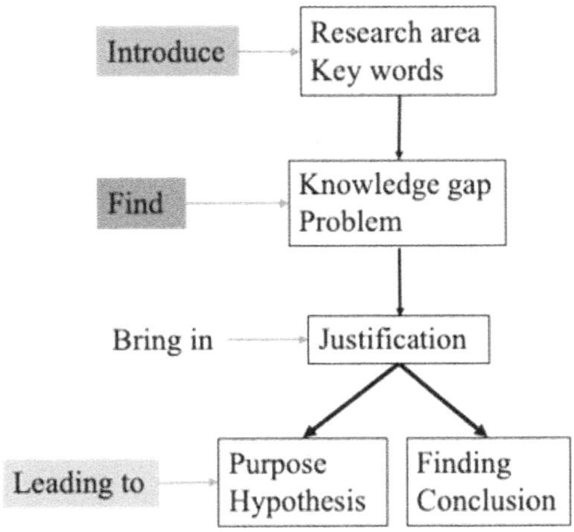

The flowchart above shows four components of an introduction.

## Research Motivation

The *research motivation* can be the impact of the disease, mechanism, or drug target identification. To start with a broad field of importance, narrow it down to focus on the research topic. Use a contrast sentence when you raise a research question.

*Example:* Approximately four million people in the USA are currently prescribed antipsychotic drugs to manage various illnesses, such as schizophrenia, bipolar disorder, depression, anxiety, dementia, insomnia, and post-traumatic stress disorder. However, obesity induced by antipsychotic drugs is a major cause of noncompliance in antipsychotic drug treatment.

Try to use recent references when reporting a fact.

## Research Gap

The research gap is an issue that has not been studied or answered. It can be a piece of knowledge, a clinical problem, or something never explored. The identified gap in the introduction should be the topic of the research paper. *Example:* The long-term side effect of the COVID-19 vaccine.

*Why is there a need to fill the research gap?* By filling this gap, we better understand the mechanism or identification of a drug target.

*How do we fill the research gap?* It depends on how the introduction is written. This may be very detailed in the entire paper's story format. *Example:* Neurons in the central nervous system have a low capacity to repair after spontaneous injury. Stimulation of axon growth is an important strategy to encourage the repair of damaged connections.

You can use transitional words connecting the known knowledge and the research gap. *Examples:*

- *Contrast:* but, however, in spite of, yet, on the other hand, or while this may be true.
- *Illustration:* thus, namely, for example, in particular, or such as.
- *Addition:* and, in addition, also, another, again, finally.
- *Time:* after, then, next, usually, another, meanwhile, at the same time, most importantly, afterward, generally, and in order to.

## The Justification States Why You Have Decided to Pursue This Aim

A research justification is needed between the topic and the aim for carrying out the research project. A topic should be broad, while the purpose or aim is specific. The justification uses information from various areas by citing previous work to support the proposed study.

The aim or hypothesis should avoid a simple announcement without justification. *Example:* We will investigate high-fat diet-induced obesity in this study. The objective is to measure gene expression levels.

## The Final Paragraph

The last paragraph of the introduction should provide the main aim, argument, and conclusion. Then, you can let readers know the paper's work, which informs the readers of the work's roadmap and what to expect.

### *Examples:*

Aim: After the literature review and research gap identification, you could point out the purposes of the project.

- This project aimed to improve cognitive function by encouraging dietary fiber intake.
- Alternatively, you may say that it was hypothesized that dietary fiber improves cognition in severely obese patients.
- The purpose of this study was to investigate COVID-19-induced lung infection.

*Work:* You could briefly describe the work as a roadmap of where the study is going.

- In this study, we investigated increased dietary fiber intake in improving cognitive function.
- Here, we characterized the obesogenic effect of drug A using a rat model.
- We subsequently investigated the inflammatory effect of drug A in the livers and guts of obese rats.

*Findings:* Here, the findings should lean toward *qualitative,* while results lean toward *quantitative.*

- This study shows that olanzapine induces weight gain in rats.
- These results identify a novel strategy or class of small molecules to enhance axon growth after its injury.
- Here, we report that antipsychotic drug A induces hyperphagia in *C. elegans* via a different mechanism from normal feeding.

*Conclusion:* You could summarize the main statements as conclusions at the end of the last paragraph of the introduction. *Examples:* In this study, we provide, demonstrate, or suggest.

- The study provides new knowledge on the mechanism of action by reducing inflammation in the brain and improving microbiota homeostasis. In this case, having brain inflammation and microbiota together form a new concept.
- Together, our results demonstrate that drug A mediates microglia on Aβ clearance, with an implication of a promising drug candidate for Alzheimer's disease treatment.

## Two examples of introductions on "Dietary-fiber on weight management for over weight."

### Excellent Introduction:

In recent years, the prevalence of overweight and obesity has escalated globally, leading to serious public health challenges. Managing weight effectively is vital for preventing a myriad of chronic diseases such as diabetes, cardiovascular disorders, and certain cancers. Dietary interventions remain the cornerstone of non-pharmacological approaches to address this concern. Among these, the role of dietary fiber has garnered significant attention due to its potential effects on satiety, metabolic rate, and gut microbiota. This research aims to elucidate the mechanistic insights and empirical evidence surrounding dietary fiber's influence on weight management in overweight individuals. A deeper understanding could pave the way for improved dietary guidelines and interventions.

**Reasoning**: This introduction starts by highlighting the global problem, providing context for the importance of the topic. It transitions seamlessly into the significance of dietary interventions and positions dietary fiber within this domain. Finally, it conveys the aim and significance of the research clearly.

**Poorly Written Introduction:**

People have been gaining a lot of weight around the world these days. There are so many reasons why, but food is a big part of it. Some people say that fiber is good for losing weight. So, this paper will look into if fiber is actually good or not. Let's see if eating more fiber can help people not be overweight."

**Reasoning**: This introduction is colloquial and lacks precision. It doesn't adequately address the gravity of the overweight issue and fails to provide context on dietary interventions as a whole. The sentence structure and phrasing are casual and lack the formal tone expected in a research paper. Additionally, the introduction doesn't specify the research's aim beyond a vague "look into," which doesn't communicate the depth or significance of the study.

## Methods

This section describes the materials you used and how you performed the research. Researchers use this section to ensure the credibility of the results. It allows the reader to understand the findings and further researchers to replicate the findings.

*Materials:* The materials are what you use in your research. These include your experiments' raw materials, equipment, and chemicals.

*Methods:* The methods are how you conduct the research, including what type of experiments used, how to perform the investigation, and how to analyze the data; therefore, it is about the research design and statistical analysis. The methods' presentation should align with the results generated through those experimental procedures. The methodology in the proposal should be detailed and thorough. You can add pictures or illustrations in flowcharts to indicate and simplify the research design. If method descriptions are already in the literature, you should refer to them without rewriting them.

## Human subjects

*Recruitment:* The recruitment methods can include open, blind, double-blind, or stratified participant allocation; the inclusion and exclusion criteria; the geography of the participants; sample size; and power calculations.

*Demographic and clinical characteristics:* A table may present the participants' information on sex, age, race, education, employment, or baseline measures.

*Participation and attrition rates:* The participation rate is the number of participants out of the number of qualified samples. The attrition rate shows the loss of participants in a study. You should also include the study time and duration.

*Patients:* The information includes the clinical assessments, recording and analyzing medical conditions and lifestyle factors, and the disease-relevant or irrelevant to the study.

An example is seen in a previous study (Chen et al., 2019).

## Experimental animals

Medical research uses experimental animals to investigate disease mechanisms and the efficiency and safety of new candidate drugs.

- *Species and strains:* The experimental animals include mice, rats, guinea pigs, and primates. Researchers should provide the details of animal species and strains. It is essential to have animal ethics approval before any experimentation.
- *Treatment:* The animal models for medical research include gene manipulation, pharmacological intervention, and dietary intervention.
- *Characteristics:* The characteristics of animal models can include sex, age, number, housing condition (temperature, lighting), and resources of the experimental animals obtained.

## Experimental Cells

Medical experiments use cell cultures derived from tissue biopsy primary cells and immortalized cell lineages. The advantage of cell research is that it is easy to use and supply at a low cost. The disadvantage is that the physiochemical environment is different from the in vivo conditions.

- *Types:* The cells include cell lines, primary cultured cells, stem cells, and gene-mutated cells.
- *Culture:* The culture includes the media and conditions used.

*Questions*: The research questions can be the difference, association, and causal effect. (1) The difference is calculated between treatments, before and after treatments, or treated versus non-treated. (2) An association is calculated to show whether or not two variables are associated with each other. (3)The causal effect is achieved by using an intervention and monitoring the outcomes.

*Groups:* The experimental groups can be between-subjects, within-subjects, or a combination of between- and within-subjects. (1) A between-subjects design can have one control group and one or two intervention groups. (2) A within-subjects design can have one or more groups with the same subject measured multiple times. (3) A combination design would be a mix of between-subjects and within-subjects.

*Variables:* The method section should clearly define independent variables, dependent variables, and covariates.

*Time sequence:* To describe the series of experiments and timelines.

*Measurements:* The method section should detail all measurement protocols. These are the laboratory, behavior, and imaging measurements.

*Instrument:* All instruments used should be clearly described.

*Approvals:* The approvals are ethical, informed consent, and biological and gene safety.

## Statistical Analyses

The statistical analysis determines the findings and quality of the presentation. Therefore, you should use the statistical analysis correctly. The statistical analysis paragraph should be the last paragraph of the methods section.

The statistical analysis should consider independent and dependent variables, control, and confounders.

The data assumptions or prerequisites are checked, including the data type, distribution normality, and transformation.

Researchers should describe all tests used in the analysis with an explanation of their rationales in detail. You will also need to include significance or confidence interval levels, post hoc tests applied, and any thresholds used. Finally, the analysis software should be described, e.g., SPSS software or GraphPad Prism.

## Things You Need to Be Aware of When You Write a Methods Section

The reader wants to know how you designed the study and obtained the data and the results. Therefore, using the passive tense and focusing on research design is more helpful. Here are three example cases.

*Follow the research design and result:* You may point out the purpose of the method. *Example:* Twenty mice were divided into two groups and fed with either a high-fat or low-fat diet for eight weeks to induce obesity. Food intake and body weight were measured once a week (research design). Blood insulin concentrations were measured using an insulin ELISA kit (Invitrogen, Australia) at the end of treatment (research design: measure, how, and when) adipose tissue was collected for further biochemical analysis (purpose). Here we fed rats a high-fat diet to induce weight gain (adding the context for the methods).

*Avoid ingredient style: Example:* Sodium chloride, biological cells, five chemicals, reaction tube, pH meter, buffer solution. A reaction tube was used to wash biological cells. Then cells were placed into 200 ml of sodium chloride solution for ten minutes and then removed from the suspension. Cells were then left at room temperature for twenty-four hours.

*Avoid story style: Example:* First, we prepared brain cells in a sodium chloride solution. Next, we washed cells and transferred them into a buffer solution. Then, we treated the cells with 200 ml of a solution containing chemicals. After that, we took out the suspension and took some photos. Using "we" too much gives an impression of a story instead of a design- or result-driven methodology.

## Results

Overall, the presentation of results needs to be systematic, logical, and comprehensive.

*What are the two types of results?* (1) incremental results, which extend previous findings or increase the knowledge further and (2) discovery, which is the first time, plays a key role, or leads to a new concept.

*What are the key elements to be covered in the result section*? (1) answer the questions raised in the introduction, (2) present the results or findings, and (3) provide a brief justification or reason for the results.

*Use appropriate descriptions for qualitative and quantitative outcomes. Example:* Quantitative results could use "increase," "decrease," "induce," "percentage," or "association." Qualitative results may use "is," "become evident," or "report evidence."

*Show the link between the result and reason:* A clear *link* between the results ȧnd reasoning is essential in the presentation. What is the critical point of justification to pursue the production of the results? What is the required method to produce the results? However, the interpretation of the result belongs to the discussion, which should not be here.

*Present a logical flow:* A logical presentation is key to allowing the reader to follow the story. Therefore, the study's primary aim should guide the flow of paragraph orders. The presentation should be logical in either a paragraph or an entire result section. A paragraph should also have a logical arrangement, with each sentence considering a way for readers to follow easily.

*Use a systematic approach:* The systematic presentation considers a system presented as a coherent body of ideas and results. This approach should start at the beginning of the research design, which can be the approach including ideas, methodology, or both. Usually, a research paper has three to five primary outcomes and one or two minor findings. In writing, you could lay out all results, work out the meaning of these findings, and rank them from the most important to least important. Write the most critical finding first and work through the remaining findings in order.

*Make sure it is comprehensive:* A comprehensive presentation means that data is solid, thorough, or complete, supporting the idea. Conversely, when the result weakly endorses the claim, the new idea claim becomes less convincing, and the research is of low quality.

The presentation styles of results are text, table, and figure. The text should cite the table and figure presented. Normally, the order of presentation is text followed by table and figure.

The text describes the result in detail, including research outcomes, reasons, contexts, and citations. Each sentence represents a portion of data, allowing individual explanation.

The figure gives a visual impression that the author wants to deliver the central ideas or findings. You may generate figures from statistical analyses, representative images, or photos.

Figures allow communication of the outcomes to readers, attracting their attention and keeping their interest.

A table can contain a large amount of data and precise numbers. The table allows the reader to understand the data through visual content, which increases the paper's readability. You may use a table instead of text when the data is too detailed or complicated, such as research participants' demographics, clinical characteristics, and biomarker measurements and the results of statistical analyses. Sometimes, it is helpful to use a table to present the trend changes in the results.

## Paragraph

A paragraph should have its purpose and a central idea, which guide the construction and arrangement of sentences.

The paragraph structure should have the topic, body, and concluding sentences. A topic sentence describes the main idea or tells the reader about the paragraph. The body sentence provides supporting evidence, data, and explanations to develop the point or idea you want to deliver. Finally, the concluding sentence completes the paragraph's idea. All information within that paragraph should link to each other and be objective.

You should be confident with the data and understand the meaning. Too often, some authors dump the data in a paragraph with disconnected information. The reader cannot work out why the information is there. Therefore, reading and citing relevant literature and making logical connections are necessary. Construct a paragraph with a logical story that readers can follow, addressing how the results are generated and how they are relevant to the question raised.

*Learn from others:* Choosing two example papers from your field as models while writing can be very helpful. You may select two high-quality papers of similar studies to yours. You can learn and follow the structure, presentation format of figures and tables, and reference citations. Action: find two papers published in your target journal and read them carefully! Do not try to create a new style at the early stage of research paper writing.

## Checklist

- Each paragraph addresses one central question only.
- Make sure that your main findings address the main questions raised at the beginning of the paper.
- Try to give a brief rationale for the results by citing a previous and critical paper.
- Describe the method name used to generate that particular result.
- Cite figures and tables as the backbone to support your results and any claims.

## Things to Avoid in the Results Section

- Do not include irrelevant results. You should present the findings because they relate to the research topic. For example, a study investigates a hormone: "Brain-Derived Neurotrophic Factor Affects Cognitive Function in Schizophrenia." The data should be blood BDNF levels and cognition scores of the patients. Others, such as liver functions, are outside the topic and should not be included unless there is a clear link.
- Avoid interpretation of the results, because this belongs to the discussion.
- Avoid vague or nonspecific phrases that rely on the reader to understand why, how, and what. The ambiguity can stifle the clarity of the paper.
- Try not to list the results alone without giving any reasons or justifications.
- Try not to start with "Table" or "Figure." For example, Based on table 1, obesity impairs glucose metabolism. It is better to say: Obesity impairs glucose metabolism (table 1).
- An extensive introduction in the results section is not necessary. Instead, it should be brief with just one or two sentences to justify why to generate the results.
- Try to avoid extensive methods or statistical analysis.
- Avoid bias. For example, selective reporting of positive and negative findings. Selective choosing of the papers which support the results.
- Do not present the results without statistical analysis. Do not include raw data.

## Examples

### Excellent Written Result Section

Participants who incorporated higher dietary-fiber into their meals demonstrated a significant reduction in weight compared to the control group ($p < 0.01$). Over a 12-week period, the high dietary-fiber group showed an average weight loss of 5.2kg ± 1.3, whereas the control group displayed an average loss of 1.0kg ± 0.5. This was further supported by a significant reduction in waist circumference in the high dietary-fiber group (mean decrease of 3.4cm) compared to the control (mean decrease of 0.8cm, $p < 0.05$). The association between dietary-fiber intake and weight loss remained significant even after adjusting for confounding variables such as physical activity and caloric intake.

### Poorly Written Result Section

People who ate more fiber lost some weight. The ones who didn't eat that much fiber didn't lose as much weight. After 12 weeks, it seemed like the fiber group lost around 5kg, maybe a bit more or less, and the other group didn't lose much. The fiber group's waists got smaller too, I think about 3cm less, and the other group's waists didn't change much. Maybe other factors like exercise affected this, but we're not sure.

**Comparisons**:

1. **Clarity**: The excellent section provides clear, precise data with statistical significance mentioned, while the poorly written section lacks detail and is ambiguous.
2. **Data Representation**: In the excellent section, data is presented using standard research terminology and includes mean values and adjustments for confounders. The poorly written section merely provides approximate values.
3. **Professionalism**: The excellent section uses a professional tone suitable for scientific research. The poorly written section uses informal language and doesn't sound scientific.
4. **Accuracy**: The excellent section considers all relevant details, ensuring results are accurate. In contrast, the poorly written section lacks this attention to detail and may leave readers questioning the validity of the results.
5. **Structure**: The excellent section is well-structured and flows logically, whereas the poorly written section jumps from one idea to another without a clear flow.

## Discussion

The discussion section serves the purpose of interpreting the results. The discussion section explains the results' meaning, while the results section is about reporting facts.

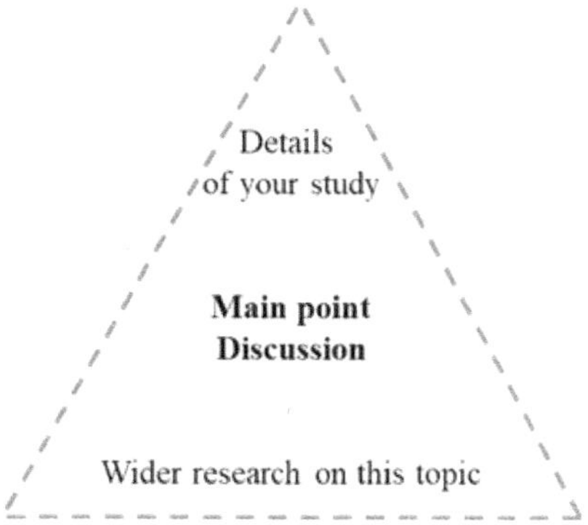


The figure shows that a rule of thumb starts with a focused point from the top of the triangle and then broadens it to form a link with what we already know. At the end of the discussion section, you could point out the weaknesses and limitations of the study and make recommendations for future research.

## Link to Existing Knowledge

The discussion allows researchers to link the new findings from the present study and the existing literature relevant to the results. The discussion section reviews the experimental details and presents the main points that can be extended to a broad field connected to the research topic.

In a discussion, a thorough literature review is essential for data interpretation. Consider the following points to have a good literature review that explains the findings.

- *Linking:* Have an overview of the field that links to the results to assist in interpreting results.
- *Similar finding:* If the results of your study are similar or match previous research, the discussion is limited to supporting and confirming the previous work. In this case, the discussion length should be relatively short.
- *Different findings:* If the results differ from previous studies, you should provide a detailed explanation or discussion. You should not leave the readers to figure out the meaning. It is common in human studies that variations can occur because of many potential confounding factors, and sometimes there is a limited sample size. Therefore, it is helpful to do a summary in the form of a literature review and point out where the results fit.
- *New finding:* If the result is new, has never been reported before, and may lead to a new concept, you will need to spend the time to develop a comprehensive discussion paragraph. This paragraph will explain why this discovery is a new concept. What is the background? What is the significance?

## The First Paragraph of the Discussion

This paragraph is usually an introductory paragraph or a summary of the key findings. Here, you should provide the main idea for performing the project without repeating the introduction. This paragraph requires a clear concept, logical order, and concluding remarks. It can also be written as a summary, briefing the reader on the key results.

## Paragraphs

Intermediate paragraphs should give your opinions in favor of or against the idea discussed, critical appraisal, and learning points. You can use previous studies to explain and emphasize your findings.

A paragraph should focus on a single significant finding or discussion point. A new finding does not mean a single result or a single picture, but it can come from several experimental results.

A discussion paragraph should have focused on the following:

- Interpreting the meaning of a finding;
- Explaining how the result fits the research topic or literature and its external validity; and
- Generating a conclusion.

It prefers to start with the most straightforward or well-accepted concept as a foundation from which you could build a complex idea.

## A Concluding Paragraph

The last paragraph of the discussion is a synthesis of the findings from the paper. In writing this paragraph, consider the following:

*Main points:* A couple of sentences provide a "take-home" message or main findings, which synthesize all the results, leading to conclusions.

*Why is this work interesting?* You may point out the project's significance and whether people could use this data to help their work, which relates to external validity.

*Limitations:* You may indicate some limits of the work. Variations and potential confounding factors are always limitations, particularly in clinical research.

*Recommendations:* Are there any recommendations for future studies?

*Key points:* This paragraph requires simplicity, clarity, and effectiveness in delivering the final remarks.

## Subtitle

A paragraph subtitle is used to highlight the main topic of that paragraph. It helps ensure that anything unrelated to the subtitle does not belong in the section. Therefore, the subtitle also helps keep the discussion focused on the main point. The subtitle should be short, a phrase or a sentence. It is preferred to use a phrase.

## Between Paragraphs

- An idea should serve as an intrinsic link between paragraphs, leading to a logical presentation.
- The sequence between the paragraphs should be conceptually clear and in a logical order.
- Although each paragraph can stand alone, it will finally *lead* to the paper's conclusion.

The below breakdown aligns each segment of the discussion sections to the respective rules, clearly illustrating the elements that differentiate a well-written section from a poorly written one.

**Excellent Written Discussion Section:**

- The findings of our study highlight a significant correlation between dietary fiber intake and weight management in overweight individuals. (1. Clarity and Structure)
- Dietary fiber has been posited to increase satiety, potentially leading to reduced energy intake (Smith et al., 2019). Our results are consistent with earlier research by Jones and colleagues (2018), who found a decrease in body weight among individuals with increased fiber consumption. (2. Connection to Previous Research)
- The mechanisms by which fiber affects weight are multifaceted, possibly involving the alteration of gut microbiota composition, thereby influencing energy regulation (White et al., 2020). (3. Mechanistic Insight)
- However, it is crucial to acknowledge potential limitations, such as the reliance on self-reported dietary intakes which might introduce recall bias. (4. Limitations)
- Future studies could delve deeper into distinguishing the effects of soluble and insoluble fibers on weight management. (5. Future Research Directions)

**Poorly Written Discussion Section:**

- So, our research showed that eating more fiber is good for weight loss for overweight people. (1. Lack of Formality)
- Some other people have also said this before like Smith and some others in 2019. (2. Ambiguity and 3. Absence of References)
- Maybe because when you eat fiber, you feel full and eat less, I think. (1. Lack of Formality and 2. Ambiguity)
- There's also something about gut bacteria or something, but not sure. (2. Ambiguity)
- Anyway, the people in our research told us what they ate but who knows if they were lying or forgetting stuff. (4. Potential Bias)
- Some other studies should maybe see if there's a difference between different types of fibers. (2. Ambiguity and 5. Lack of Forward-Thinking)

**Excellent Conclusion and Significance:**

Conclusion and Significance: Our research elucidates the pivotal role of dietary fiber in weight management for overweight individuals. Incorporating fiber-rich foods not only curbed appetite but significantly influenced weight loss. Emphasizing dietary fiber could revolutionize approaches to weight management in this population, offering a sustainable, natural intervention.

Comments: This conclusion is concise, directly ties the main findings (curbing appetite and influencing weight loss) to the topic (dietary fiber's role in weight management), and speaks to the larger implications (revolutionizing weight management approaches).

**Poorly Written Conclusion and Significance:**

Conclusion and Significance: So, in our study, we found out that if overweight people eat more fiber, they might lose some weight. I guess fiber is kind of important for these people, and maybe others should look into it too. It's a good thing.

Comments: This version is informal, lacks specific findings, doesn't provide a clear link between dietary fiber and its significance in weight management, and uses ambiguous phrases like "kind of" and "I guess," which undermines the credibility and strength of the findings.

## Things to Avoid When Writing the Discussion

- Do not repeat the introduction. The discussion is about the interpretation of the results.
- Do not repeat the results in the discussion.
- Try not to use numbers, as the numbers belong to the result section. Instead, the discussion should lean toward being qualitative and interpretative.
- Do not raise too many speculations without supporting data. There must be supporting data, either from the study or the literature.
- Try to end the discussion without leaving the reader "hanging." The conclusion should not be left for the reader to figure out.
- Do not cite unrelated literature or irrelevant information.

## Checklist of a Discussion Section

- The discussion should cover all hypotheses proposed in the introduction section.
- The discussion should interpret the results or findings.
- Usually, the discussion section should have three to five main points. These points are based on the results and are placed in the same order.
- The order should start with the critical findings and leave the negative or controversial results to the later part of the discussion.

## Paper Submission

*Choice of the Journal:* Field of relevance: clinical or basic. The level of impact factor. You may find a list of journals on Web of Science.

*Cover letter to the editor:* (1) Explain the work, but do not oversell. (2) Point out the novelty and critical points. (3) Highlight the significance of the work. (4) Always suggest referees, but try not to use "best friends."

*Selection of reviewers:* (1) The reviewer should be able to understand your work. (2) You should not use your best friends as reviewers. The work relevance is more appropriate. (3) Try to suggest experienced researchers.

*Revision:* Revisions include *acceptable, minor revision, major revision,* or *rejection.* It is best to treat criticisms and suggestions constructively. Carefully respond to all questions point by point. Write a letter to the editor to acknowledge the editor's and reviewers' work.

## Science Citation Index

The Institute for Scientific Information (ISI, US) produced the science citation index (SCI)). Launched in 1964, SCI is the most extensive database that holds the most authoritative papers. It collects from all fields of science, >171 majors, and ~8,500 journals from 1900 to the present. It is available online, e.g., Web of Science.

## Journal Impact Factor

The journal impact factor is the number of journal citations divided by the total number of papers that the journal has published in the previous two years. You can find a journal's impact factor online: Journal Citation Reports (JCR):

https://clarivate.com/webofsciencegroup/solutions/journal-citation-reports/.

## How Is the Journal Impact Factor Calculated?

*Example:* A journal has two hundred papers cited one thousand times in the previous two years (e.g., from 2013 to 2014). The impact factor is 1000/200 = 5.

Possible uses of the impact factor: (1) Editors and publishers use SCI to chart the growth of citations of their journals and their competitors'. (2) Researchers use SCI to monitor where their research papers might obtain the most attention. (3) Some university recruitment and promotion committees use SCI to evaluate the quality of the research papers published by current employees. (4) Some government agencies use SCI to measure the quality of research papers published. (5) Some competitive funding bodies use SCI to evaluate the quality of journal papers published by potential grant recipients.

## What Is the H-Index?

The h-index was first suggested in 2005 by Jorge Hirsch, a physicist at the University of California San Diego. The h-index measures both the productivity and impact of a scientist's/scholar's research.

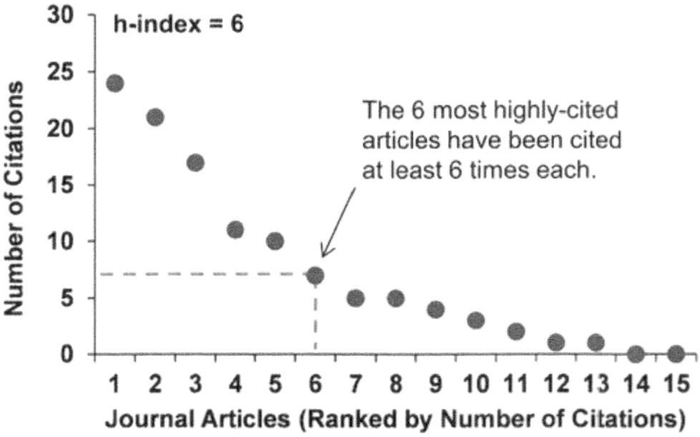


For example, an h-index of 6 means that an author has six papers cited at least six times. You can find a researcher's h-index on Web of Science, Scopus, and Google Scholar.

**ASK YOURSELF**

What are the essential criteria for a research paper?
What are the standard structures of a research paper?
What are the key elements of constructing a good title?
What is a structured or unstructured abstract?
What should you tell readers in the introduction?
What should you present in the materials and methods section?
What are the key elements to be covered in the result section?
When do you choose to use the text, figure or table in the result section?
What is the purpose of the discussion section?
What are the differences between conclusion and significance?

CHAPTER 4

# Review Paper

**TOPIC OUTLINE**

Narrative review
General review
Systematic review
Meta-analysis

Today, a professional worker or researcher needs to review the literature regularly. The information develops rapidly, with more than thirty thousand papers per year or one hundred papers a day. Therefore, it is vital to keep updated with new knowledge, irrespective of how many years you have worked in the field. A review paper should address a specific topic in the past, present, and future. In addition, it should evaluate the quality of the research papers.

## Aims

A review paper aims to review recent progress in a particular topic concisely. Overall, a review paper should summarize and analyze the existing documents in the literature, comment on the previous findings, provide new insights, interpret a topic through thorough and systematic evaluation, and generate new ideas. It can have multiple purposes:

- To get a comprehensive understanding of the research field or professional area topic.
- To inform the researcher or professional worker about their topic's past, current, and future directions.

- To understand the discrepancies and controversial issues in the field.
- To develop an opinion based on reading and analysis.
- To develop a meaningful and focused research project.

## Structure

A review paper has a similar structure as a research paper but differs in content and emphasis.

The structures are the title, abstract, introduction, methods, results, discussion, conclusion, and references.

The methods section should describe the search engine used, such as PubMed, Medline, and Web of Science. The result section can include text, tables, and figures to synthesize and emphasize the information.

## Focused Topic

A review paper needs to have a well-defined scope and focus as the review topic.

You may provide a comprehensive knowledge foundation and *summarize* current thinking on the topic. Also, you could highlight the relevant methodologies and research techniques.

## Area's Advancement and Shortfalls

- A review needs to point out new information and recent advances. These will be the bases and highlights to build up the review paper.
- A review should identify *gaps*, point out *hot spots*, and raise *frontline questions* for critical comments.

## Conclusion and Impact

- A review should lead to *innovative conclusions* from the existing data. You may synthesize, rather than segregate, the current findings from various papers to support a new idea.
- A review should highlight the impacts of the critical points reviewed, including the field, fundamental, clinical, or social impact research.
- Finally, a review should suggest potential research areas and explore *future* directions.

## Review Paper Types

*Narrative review:* A narrative review summarizes a specific topic, comments on the literature's pros and cons, and provides new ideas.

*Systematic review:* A systematic review uses systematic methods to find and evaluate all relevant research.

*Mata-analysis:* A meta-analysis builds statistics into the review.

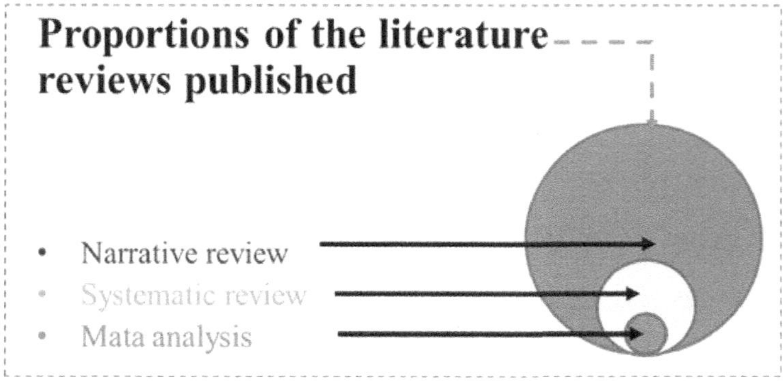


The above figure shows the types of literature reviews, including narrative review, systematic review, and meta-analysis. The proportions are that the narrative review is the most common, followed by systematic review and meta-analysis.

## Narrative Review

A *narrative review* is an evidence-based summary outlining and commenting on a specific topic. It focuses on an issue and understands what is happening in the literature, covering several particular questions. There are many more focused narrative or specific topic review papers than other literature review papers. The narrative review includes general, theoretical, methodological, and historical reviews.

## General Review

A *general review* paper aims to review recent or current progress in a particular topic. Generally, the article summarizes the current knowledge of the topic; therefore, it frequently attracts a broad range of readers. Because there is a demand for understanding the topic, the review introduces and discusses the findings reported in recent research articles.

*Key points:* Broad interest, precise aim, and comprehensive literature.

*Impact:* In the preparation stage, the author should consider who will be interested in the topic and how extensive this readership will likely be. Is the review likely to have a high impact? What will be the scope of the science? What should the emphasis be? Here, we have three general review papers.

- A Comprehensive Review on Metabolic Syndrome (Kaur, 2014).
- Antipsychotic-Induced Weight Gain (Kaur, 2014).
- Inflammatory Cytokines and Antipsychotic-Induced Weight Gain (Fonseka et al., 2016).

Up to 2022, the first paper attracted 2,378 citations, the second one attracted 903 citations, and the third one attracted 65 citations. The impact size is predictable when you decide on the topic or title of the review. Clearly, the scope that reflects the number of readers is the greatest in the first paper, followed by the second and then the third paper. Therefore, the first paper has attracted more citations than others, although this does not mean the third paper is less important scientifically.

**Theoretical Review**

A *theoretical literature review* focuses on how the theory *develops*, *influences*, and *shapes* the research topic. It focuses on theory or mechanistically based questions.

Usually, studying the mechanism is based on cell-based and animal-based research with implications for human health; therefore, it is essential to cover all preclinical studies when searching for relevant papers in the literature. It is challenging to do mechanistic studies in a clinical trial or human research. Here, we have four theoretical review papers:

"Obesity and Cancer Mechanisms Underlying Tumour Progression and Recurrence" (Park et al., 2014).

"Obesity, the PI3K/AKT Signal Pathway, and Colon Cancer" (Huang and Chen, 2009).

"The Role of Ghrelin Signalling in Second-Generation Antipsychotic-Induced Weight Gain" (Zhang et al., 2013).

"Effects of Antipsychotic Drugs on Neurites Relevant to Schizophrenia Treatment" (Huang and Song, 2019).

Up to 2022, the citations from the first to the fourth papers were 532, 242, 55, and 28 times. The scope that reflects the number of readers is the greatest in the first paper, followed by the second, third, and fourth. Therefore, the first paper has attracted more citations than others, although this does not mean the last article is not essential scientifically.

This outcome of the citation difference should be predictable from the titles. The keywords used in the title attract readers, which should be considered in the design of a review paper.

Methodological review

A *methodological review* focuses on the methods. It can be *techniques, instruments or methodological choices* used in the studies. The review should highlight these features' strengths and weaknesses and future applications.

A methodological review can attract high citations if it has a broad audience and is helpful for general practice.

***Examples:***

- *Choice of drug delivery:* The review paper "Oral Versus Depot Antipsychotic Drugs for Schizophrenia: A Critical Systematic Review and Meta-Analysis of Randomised Long-Term Trials" has attracted more than 496 citations up to 2022 (Leucht et al., 2011).

- *Choice of research design:* Is a nonrandomized intervention an acceptable method to study child obesity prevention? In this case, the research design needs to be able to answer the research question. A review can summarize and analyze previous papers and make suggestions.
- *Instrument application:* Researchers can review an instrument's strengths, weaknesses, advancement and applications. *Example:* Magnetic resonance imaging (MRI) application in understanding human movement control.
- *Diagnostic method:* Many diagnostic ways are continuously advancing. A review can help practitioners use advanced diagnostic tools and method developers to know the future direction. *Example:* The polymerase chain reaction: current and future applications.

### Historical Review

A historical review aims to document how science has evolved over a long period. It often starts with the first-time event and then follows on from there. It can be a medical condition or issue, concept, symptom, or theory. *Example:* A historical review paper, "Another View of the History of Antipsychotic Drug Discovery and Development" (Carpenter and Davis, 2012), attracted eighty-five citations over the last ten years. Normally, only reviewing history does not attract many citations. Solving the current issues will attract more readers to cite your work.

## Checklist of a Narrative Review Paper

- *Scope and focus:* First is to define the scope and focus of the review paper, considering the precision and external validity.
- *Summary foundation:* You can start by presenting current knowledge and ideas, laying a comprehensive foundation on the topic.
- *Impact:* You may address the implications of the review topic in the field, clinical, or social aspects to make sure that the subject links to the readers.
- *New information:* You should provide the latest news and recent advances in the topic. These points will be the highlights of the review. Usually, an established area has the information that can be drawn after the analysis.
- *Gaps and hot spots:* Identify gaps, hot spots, and frontline questions. These points allow you to make comments. For example, what are the controversial issues, and why are they controversial? Is there any missing information?
- *New ideas:* Has the review's analysis generated new opinions or innovative conclusions? Using the strategy of analyzing relevant papers supports the new ideas and conclusions. The review should include the process of how you did the analysis.
- *Methodology:* You may highlight the primary methods and research techniques used in the field.
- *Limitations:* What are the limits? You could point out why this is limited if there is an unsolved problem.

- *Future:* Suggest potential research areas to explore future directions. Where is the improvement required or needed in future research? What is the future direction of this research?

## Systematic Review

A systematic review uses a systematic and reproducible approach to identify, evaluate, and synthesize available data under a research question or topic. A systematic review does the following:

- Systematically searches for all relevant studies.
- Critically appraises and selects all relevant studies.
- Extracts, synthesizes, and analyzes data.
- Presents and interprets data.

**A systematic review is a review:**

- Of a clearly formulated question
- To systematically search for relevant studies
- To critically appraise and select all relevant studies
- To extract, synthesize and analyze data
- To present and interpret data

**Protocol of meta-analysis**

Defining the review question
↓
Searching for papers
↓
Selecting the papers
↓
To extract, synthesize, and analyze data
↓
Interpretation of the results

Here are the critical points on the left and a chart on the right applied in a systematic review.

A systematic review is usually broader than a narrative review. It requires a great deal of time and work. Usually, the review should not miss any papers from the last twenty years if they fit specific inclusion/exclusion criteria.

## Advantages of a Systematic Review

*Synthesis of all data:* A systematic review provides overall and complete evidence of the data under a research topic or question. Usually, it should be thorough, covering a broad scope and extensive history. A systematic review follows a standard structure in collecting and analyzing the data. Therefore, the data collection should be highly standardized and complete. A systematic review can help researchers and clinicians make informed decisions and have up-to-date knowledge.

*Minimization of bias:* Since a systematic review uses a standardized protocol to determine which articles should be included (selection criteria), it minimizes the bias.

*Conflicts between papers:* It is often difficult to judge which conclusion is correct when there are conflicting findings among studies. Inconsistent results often arise when the study has a small sample size or is a retrospective study. In this case, a review of all available papers is essential.

*Research question:* A systematic review can address the following questions: (1) *Association:* Is one treatment more effective than another? In this case, case-control and cohort studies are used. (2) *Causal:* Will exposure to an agent result in disease? In this case, intervention studies or well-designed longitudinal cohort studies are used.

*Literature search and data extraction:* The literature search is a critical step and often is the most challenging part of a systematic review. The literature review process needs to be comprehensive. The information reviewed must be up to date.

*Searching tools:* There are many searching tools, including (1) PubMed, Web of Science, Medline, and Scopus; (2) EMBASE and CINAHL; (3) unpublished clinical trials; (4) Cochrane Central Register of Controlled Trials.

*Data used for a systematic review:* It is necessary to know what kind of data is more valid than others when collecting data for a systematic review. Systematic review often uses the data from randomized controlled trials, cohort studies, and case-control studies. However, randomized controlled trials are more rigorous than cohort and case-control studies. Therefore, a review based on well-designed randomized controlled trials will likely be more valid and accurate than a review based on other study types.

*Data synthesis:* After you have extracted the data and assessed its quality and validity, the outcomes of individual studies are pooled and presented as a summary indicating the results or effects.

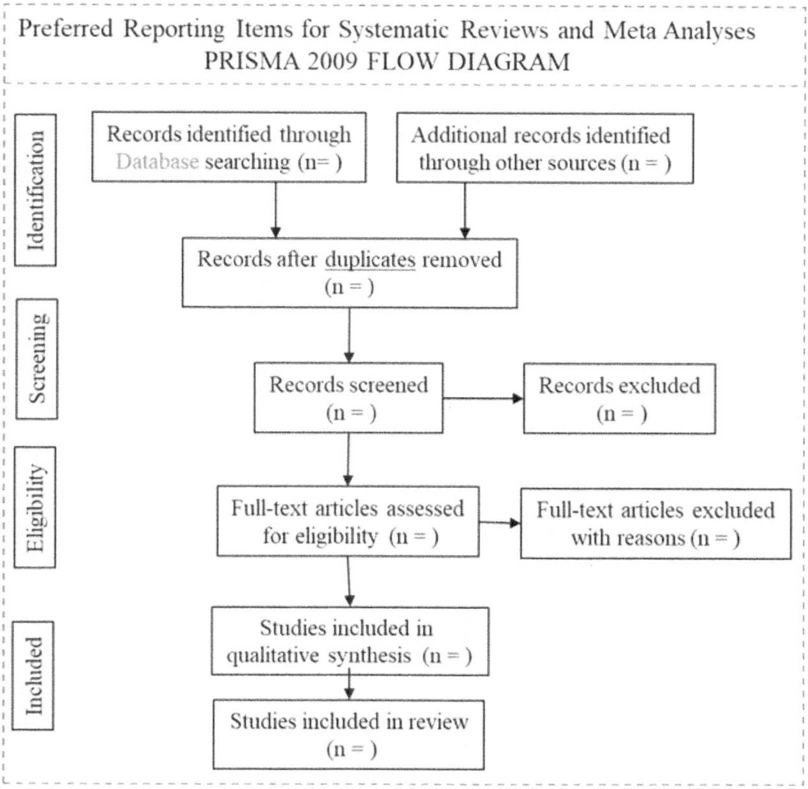


The flowchart shows "Preferred Reporting Items for Systematic Reviews and Meta-Analyses, PRISMA 2009." PRISMA is a structured search for systematic reviews and meta-analyses. PRISMA can use the data from randomized trials and other intervention studies. First, the papers related to the topic are identified by searching databases. After collecting the articles, researchers identify which articles can be used based on the systematic review and meta-analysis inclusion and exclusion criteria. Once eligibility has been determined, the papers are used. So when writing a systematic review, you may follow the Preferred Reporting Items for Systematic Reviews and Meta-Analyses (PRISMA) guideline.

## Meta-Analysis

A *meta-analysis* is a statistical technique that combines similar but independent studies to estimate a treatment or association effect. Virtually all meta-analyses are based on a systematic review. However, not all systematic reviews must have a meta-analysis.

To ensure a thorough and consistent outcome, you should have a standard protocol to identify all the relevant papers. It is noted that only some data or papers are qualified to be used in a meta-analysis.

Aims

- To use analytical or statistical methods for a systematic review.
- To estimate the overall treatment or association effects.
- To explore heterogeneity or variations between studies. If there are differences between studies, the salient question is how much difference there is.
- To assess publication bias and the quality of the research papers.

Data Types

The data used in a meta-analysis can either be dichotomous or continuous (see the table below). It requires that the data focuses on the effect measurement. Dichotomous data is binary and used to calculate the odds ratio, relative risk, and risk difference. Continuous data is used to calculate the mean and standardized mean differences.

**The types of data used in meta-analysis**

*It requires the data focusing on effect measurement.*

<table>
<tr><th>Type of data</th><th colspan="6">Outcome measure</th></tr>
<tr><td>Dichotomous (binary, displayed in 2X2 table)</td><td colspan="2">Odds ratio (OR)</td><td colspan="2">Relative risk (RR)</td><td colspan="2">Risk difference (RD)</td></tr>
<tr><td>Continuous</td><td colspan="3">Mean difference (MD)</td><td colspan="3">Standardized mean difference (SMD)</td></tr>
</table>

*Search papers for meta-analysis:* The title of a research paper can be used as the first screen to determine if an article may be included in a meta-analysis.

*Example:* A paper's title is "High-Intensity Training Leads to Better Glucose Control Than Moderate-Intensity Training in Type 2 Diabetes Patients." This paper has addressed PICO(T) criteria; therefore, it will likely be used in a meta-analysis. PICO(T) refers to patients with type 2 diabetes (P), high-intensity interval training (I), moderate to intensity training (C), glucose metabolism control (e.g., Hb1Ac, FBG) (O). The title did not mention the time (T).

*Outcome metrics:* Data from the literature often uses *different* outcome metrics, making combining the data awkward. Therefore, you may have to convert the data to a *uniform* metric for data pooling.

## Data Not to Be Included:

- Data should not be combined if there are conflicting and widely variable data.
- If the data is very unusual, you should not include that data. *Example:* if the data has a standard deviation that is too small or too large.

**Statistical software:** Meta-analysis requires computer software for data synthesis and analysis. (1) Free software: RevMan 5.3: from Cochrane Collaboration; EpiMeta: from Epi Info. (2) Paid software: Meta module in STATA and others.

## Forest Plot

A *forest plot* displays estimated results from multiple research papers addressing the same question. Therefore, it is a pooled evaluation of an effect combining numerous individual investigations. Since some studies contribute more to the pooled estimate, these studies will give more weight. The amount of weight given often relies on the sample size and standard deviation. A forest plot can use either dichotomous or continuous data.

## What Does a Forest Plot Provide?

- The effect estimates of each study using mean difference, frequency, OR, and RR.
- The 95% CI of each study indicates homogeneity.
- An overall effect is a summary of all papers shown graphically and numerically.
- A visual appraisal of heterogeneity.

## Fixed Effects Model

The *fixed effects model* assumes that the true effect of treatment is the same for every study. It is used when the test shows data homogeneity: $p > 0.05$, $I^2 < 25\%$.

## Random Effects Model

The *random effects model* assumes that the true effect estimate for each study varies. It is used when the test shows data heterogeneity: $p < 0.05$, $I^2$ is ≥ 25%.

## Heterogeneity

*Heterogeneity* is the scope of inconsistency between the effect evaluation and multiple papers. Here the $p$ and $I^2$ values are relevant. The $p$-value represents the probability of rejecting the null hypothesis when it is true. The $I^2$ value indicates the size of the heterogeneity. A forest plot shows an overall effect of heterogeneity using the $p$-value from a Z test.

## $X^2$ test

- A high $p$-value suggests homogeneity, $p > 0.05$.
- A low $p$-value suggests heterogeneity, $p < 0.05$.

## $I^2$

- 25% indicates low heterogeneity
- 50% indicates moderate heterogeneity
- 75% indicates high heterogeneity.

## Geometrics

*Square:* The square depicts the effect of a single study, and the size is proportional to the weighting.

*Horizontal line:* indicates the confidence interval (CI 95%). The shorter the CI, the smaller the variation and the more accurate the effect evaluation.

*Vertical line:* indicates no effect (0 in a continuous variable plot, 1 in a binary variable plot). If the horizontal line (CI) crosses the vertical line, it indicates no statistical significance. Otherwise, there is a statistical difference.

*Diamond:* The diamond depicts the pooled effect. The center of the diamond is the point estimate, and the width is the CI.

*Forest plot of the outcome with dichotomous and homogeneous data*

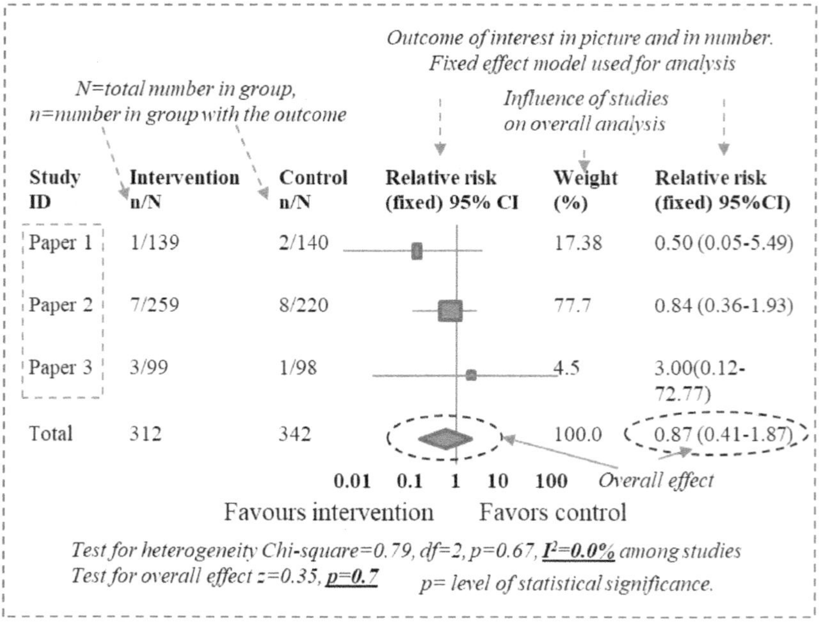


## ***The plot has six columns:***

- The first column shows the study ID. The ID can be the author's name and year of publication. (Here, we used papers 1, 2, and 3.)
- The second and third columns are the intervention and control groups. The lowercase *n* refers to the subject

number in the group with the outcome. The uppercase *N* refers to the total number of subjects in the group.

- The fourth column has a line of no effect. The vertical line indicates there is no effect. If the symbol is to the left of the line, the results favor the intervention over the control. If the symbol is to the right of the line, the results favor the control over the intervention. The sample size and standard deviation have a combined effect that contributes to the overall effect. In this example, the overall effect of $p = 0.7$ is $> 0.05$; therefore, it is statistically insignificant. It can also be seen in the plot, with the overall effect (diamond symbol) overlapping the line of no effect.
- The fifth column indicates the weight (%).
- The sixth column is outcomes in numeric form.

*Heterogeneity:* Another aspect is the chi-square test. The degree of freedom is two because there are three groups; $p = 0.67$, $>$ 0.05, indicating no heterogeneity. It can also be seen when looking at the plot. The data are homogeneous. Since the data are homogeneous, a meta-analysis uses a fixed model.

## Forest Plot of the Outcome with Continuous Variable

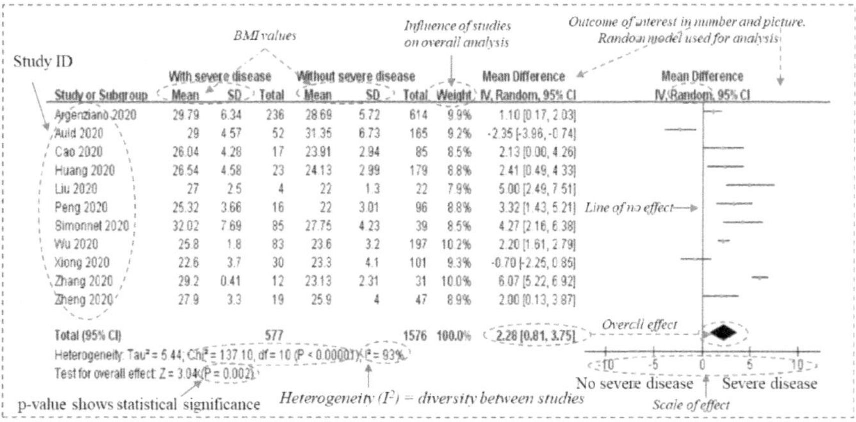


A forest plot presents the mean and standard deviation when using continuous data. The forest plot shows the mean differences in body mass index (BMI) between COVID-19 patients with and without severe disease (Chu et al., 2020).

The chi-square test yielded that $X^2$ = 123.10, df = 10, $p$ < 0.00001 and $I^2$ 93%, indicating that the data is highly heterogeneous. Therefore, a random test was used.

The analysis showed an overall effect with a $p$-value of 0.002. Therefore, there was a statistically significant mean difference in BMI between COVID-19 patients with and without severe disease. As indicated, the diamond is away from the vertical no-effect line. The overall effect is 2.28, CI 95%, 0.81–3.75.

## Forest Plot of a Binary Outcome

The study hypothesized that type 2 diabetes is a risk factor for COVID-19 severity (Pinto and Bertoluci, 2020).

The OR was used to estimate the risk factor and was calculated based on binary outcomes. The OR was the odds of an event occurring given a particular exposure relative to the odds of that same event occurring without the exposure.

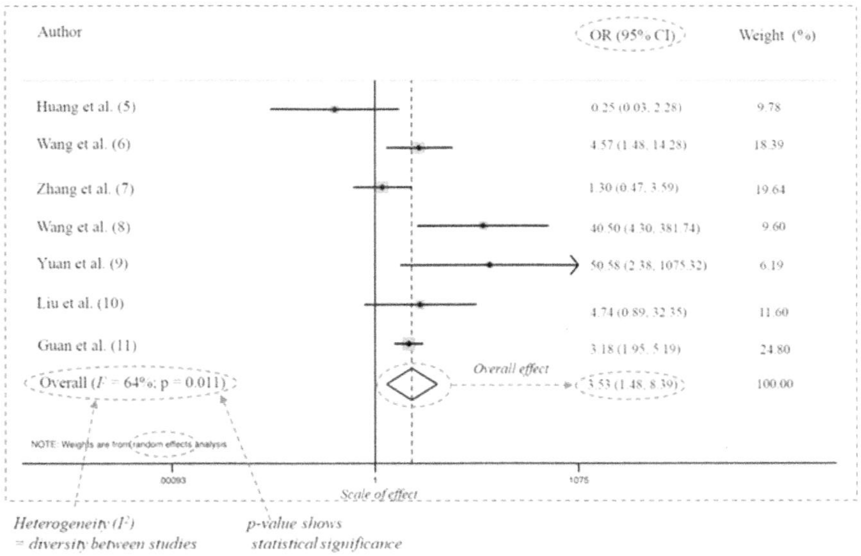


The forest plot shows the association between type 2 diabetes and the severity of COVID-19 based on seven descriptive studies.

Overall, the plot showed that the severity risk was 3.53 (95% CI, 1.48, 8.39) times higher in diabetes patients than in controls.

The data had an $I^2$ of 64% with a *p*-value of 0.011, suggesting a high heterogeneity; therefore, the analysis used a random test.

The high heterogeneity suggests that other factors could contribute to the higher risk.

## Funnel Plot

A *funnel plot* estimates publication bias and is commonly used in meta-analyses. It shows whether there is a preference for positive or negative results.

The small studies scatter widely at the bottom, and the significant effects of the large-sized studies are toward the top of the plot.

Funnel plot asymmetry indicates the heterogeneity of the studies. It reports if there is bias.

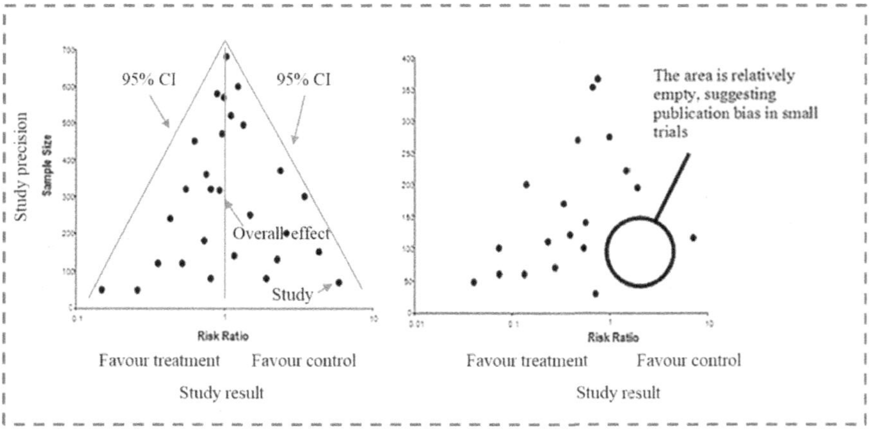


In the figure, an area gap can be seen in the right funnel plot. This area gap indicates a potential publication bias. Data is missing in the range of ~50 to 200 sample size and ~2 to 8 risk ratio.

*Example:* A systematic review and meta-analysis using mean differences to show the effects.

Most antipsychotics can induce weight gain and metabolic complications. Several randomized trials have shown metformin to be effective in prevention, but this still hasn't been included in clinical guidelines on managing antipsychotic-induced weight gain.

The research design is to use randomized controlled trials assessing metformin's efficacy in treating antipsychotic-induced weight gain (de Silva et al., 2016). The search includes the Cochrane Central Register of Controlled Trials and MEDLINE from 2000 to 2015. The magnitude of heterogeneity was determined using the $I^2$ statistic. Meta-analysis was carried out using the random effects model, as the data were heterogeneous. Statistical analysis was performed using Review Manager version 5.2.

Meta-analysis of twelve studies found that treatment with metformin resulted in significantly more weight loss than placebo in patients treated with antipsychotics [-3.27 kg (95 % CI −4.66 to −1.89) ($Z = 4.64$, $p < 0.001$)].

There was significant heterogeneity among the studies ($p < 0.001$, $I^2 = 82\%$).

The funnel plot showed no evidence of asymmetry of metformin versus placebo for treatment of antipsychotic-induced weight gain ($p = 0.662$).

It was concluded that metformin was effective in treating antipsychotic-induced weight gain in patients with schizophrenia or schizoaffective disorder.

*Example: Literature review.* Here is an example of a literature review. The title of this literature review is "The Role of Ghrelin

Signaling in Second-Generation Antipsychotic-Induced Weight Gain" (Zhang et al., 2013). This paper is a narrative review on antipsychotic drugs affecting the hunger hormone ghrelin signaling in the brain. It is known that second-generation antipsychotic drugs increase weight gain and obesity and are associated with metabolic disorders. However, the mechanism is not clear. Ghrelin is the only hunger hormone in the peripheral tissue that regulates food intake. Previously, it was thought that patients on second-generation antipsychotic drugs had increased ghrelin. Currently, the data are inconsistent due to human sample variations and the difficulty in precisely measuring food intake. This review collected, integrated, and analyzed the data from human, rodent, and cell literature. A new conclusion was generated that ghrelin is a potential new drug target for treating second-generation antipsychotic drug-induced obesity and its associated metabolic disorders.

**ASK YOURSELF**

What are the three main types of review papers?
What are the emphases of a general review, theoretical review, methodological review, and historical review?
What is a systematic review?
What are the advantages of a systematic review?
What kind of data is preferred in a systematic review?
What does PRISMA mean?
What are the aims of a meta-analysis?
What type of data should a meta-analysis not use?
What can a forest plot tell you?
What is the heterogeneity reported in a meta-analysis?
What can a funnel plot tell you?

CHAPTER 5

# Other Papers

**TOPIC OUTLINE**

Brief communication
Commentary
Perspective
Conference abstract

## Brief Communication

A brief communication or rapid communication is an independent report describing a valuable contribution to the research field of timely importance.

A portion of a research study can be published if the entire experiment cannot be completed in a given time. You can publish a brief communication that is a part of the whole study. The downside of this is you cannot publish the same results again because a short communication is considered a publication.

*Some considerations when writing a brief communication are as follows:*

- It reports novel and exciting but incomplete (a brief communication) or preliminary (a rapid communication) results. It can also be a report on negative outcomes or different opinions.
- A brief communication is time and manner sensitive. Usually, there are some novel observations, but no

mechanism is known to underline the statement. It has some similarities to a nonstructured abstract.

- The content should be attractive to other researchers and could stimulate follow-up studies. It will be short and provide key points to the reader.
- It can also be a case report or case series report, which are considered short communications because the work is incomplete.

*Example:* Brief communication. Here is an example of a brief communication published in the journal *Schizophrenia Research*. The title of this paper is "Serum NCAM Levels and Cognitive Deficits in First-Episode Schizophrenia" (An et al., 2018). Why was this paper published as a brief communication instead of a full research paper? This work is a typical association study between serum NCAM molecule levels and cognition in schizophrenia with no underlying mechanism investigated. The researcher investigated a single time point examining the differences in plasma NCAM levels and cognitive functions between patients and healthy controls. To qualify for a full research paper, it will require a full story, but at the present stage, the research is incomplete. A possible full report can be: (1) an extension of the NACM system with multiple biomarkers investigated, (2) providing an NCAM intervention study using animal models, or (3) possible underlying mechanisms of an increased NCAM in the patients, such as genetic factors. The hypothesis can be developed based on the results of this short communication.

## Commentary

A commentary is a short article providing critical views or comments on a recently published paper, book, or report. Usually, the author is an expert in the field, giving the *interpretation*, *evaluation*, and *opinion* on the original article.

- *New idea:* The commentator may provide new ideas based on the original paper and appraise the new concept presented in the article.
- *Criticism:* It aims to improve the research.
- *A call to action:* It emphasizes the implication of the results beyond what has been mentioned in the paper.
- *Time:* It would be best within three months of publishing the original paper.
- *Significance:* A commentary may highlight several points of broader relevance to the field. For example, how to apply the findings to human health.

*Example: Commentary.* Here is an example of a commentary paper. The title is "Comment On: Oleanolic Acid Co-Administration Alleviates Ethanol-Induced Hepatic Injury Via Nrf-2 and Ethanol-Metabolizing Modulation in Rats" (Camer and Huang, 2014a). This short commentary article has commented on a lack of studying the involvement of NF-κB. If the study had investigated NF-κB, it would have helped to understand the mechanism by which oleanolic acid reduces IL-6 and Nrf in alcohol-induced hepatic oxidative stress and inflammation.

## Perspective

A *perspective* should present the author's *opinion*, a *new viewpoint*, and *some data* on existing problems and concepts on a specific topic.

*Focus:* A perspective focuses on a topic's current and future direction.

*Viewpoints:*

- A specific topic based on an existing problem.
- A fundamental concept or general concept.
- An innovation.

A perspective article is usually between 1,500 and 3,000 words (including abstract, main text, references, and figure legends).

*Example: Perspective.* Here is an example of a perspective article (Camer and Huang, 2014b). The title is "The Endothelin Pathway: A Protective or Detrimental Target of Bardoxolone Methyl on Cardiac Function in Patients with Advanced Chronic Kidney Disease," published in the journal *Nephrology*. Bardoxolone methyl shows promise in treating obesity and metabolic disorders. However, recent clinical trial reports reveal that this compound can cause cardiovascular events in patients with chronic kidney disease. There is much confusion and conflicting perspectives on whether this compound is likely to become a clinical drug in the future. This article points out that further investigation is required to determine a specific receptor ($EF_A$) in the heart before a conclusion can be made to cease or further develop this candidate compound.

## Conference Abstract

A medical *conference abstract* includes five components: title and author information, introduction, methods, results, and conclusions.

*Title and author information:* The title should summarize the abstract and appear that the topic is exciting, influential, innovative, and relevant to the conference. To generate a title, select three to five keywords and string them into several sentences. You will use the sentence as the title that conveys the meaning of the work. Next, list all authors' names and their institutional affiliations.

*Introduction:* Start by outlining the question addressed by the research. Try to make the first sentence as exciting and important as possible. For example, "3.7% of the population suffer from dementia" is more appealing than "A critical cause of dementia is mental stress." Then, cite the authority paper, write what is known and what remains unknown, and lead your study to fill the knowledge gap. Finally, you can describe the purpose of the study.

*Methods:* Provide minimal sentences for readers to judge the validity of the work. An abstract may describe the research design, patient, in vivo or in vitro model information, intervention, measurements, and outcome variables.

*Results:* This consists of the most significant outcome variables compared to controls. Numerical results should include standard deviations or 95% confidence intervals and the level of the p-value for statistical significance. If the results are not statistically significant, you may give the β value indicating the power of your study to avoid possible type II errors.

*Conclusion:* One or two sentences provide the conclusion and its implications. All conclusions need data to support them. Do not present personal speculations. You may point out the generalizability or external validity of the findings.

*Improvements:* Reading the abstract aloud is an excellent way to improve logical flow and catch grammatical errors and word omissions.

*Abbreviation and jargon:* Try to reduce the use of medical jargon and excessive abbreviations to no more than three. Always spell out the abbreviations the first time they appear.

## Conference Poster Design

A *conference poster* presents the research information in a paper poster that other researchers can view. It has a short title, an introduction, experiments, results, discussion, and an acknowledgment. All writing should be brief and precise. Usually, a poster has many graphs and pictures. Refer to the instructions given by the conference committee for poster size.

*Title:* The title should be brief, exciting, and precise.

*Abstract:* Usually, a poster does not need an abstract; however, if it is required, keep it as brief as possible.

*Introduction:* Use the absolute minimum of background information and justifications.

*Materials and methods:* Briefly describe experimental equipment and procedure. Use figures and flowcharts to illustrate the experimental design. Mention the statistical analyses used and how they allowed you to address the hypothesis.

*Results:* Briefly describe qualitative and descriptive results. Present data analysis. Refer to supporting charts or images. Provide engaging figure legends that *could* stand on their own. Opt for figures over tables whenever possible.

*Conclusions:* Try to convince the visitor why the outcome is interesting. Add a sentence on future directions of research.

*Literature* cited as necessary.

*Acknowledgments:* Thank contributors and funding bodies.

*Things not to do:* Don't be too wordy or leave too much empty space.

# PART THREE
# Research Thesis

## Overview

Executive summary: A thesis is a document submitted by high-degree candidates for an academic degree, such as honors, master's, or PhD. It describes the research rationales, methods, findings, discussions, and conclusions. A thesis is a large document with a substantial degree of complexity; it explains the workflow in reaching the conclusions.

Reading and evaluating a thesis gives you a feeling about the candidate's research ability. These abilities include conducting research, analyzing the literature, presenting study designs and results, and linking the topic with the broader field.

*Thesis structure:* A typical research thesis has two to four chapters of original work sandwiched between a literature review chapter and a general discussion chapter. Usually, a PhD thesis has four, a master's has three, and an honors thesis has two experimental chapters.

*Continuity:* A thesis should provide the research project's complete and coherent story. The content should not appear disjointed, and the argument should flow logically throughout the presentation. To achieve this, you may add supporting commentary such as a foreword or summary statement at the beginning of each chapter to establish the link to previous chapters and explain how it relates to the overall thesis statement.

*Integration:* An integration is about connections between ideas, findings, and discussions. The writing requires an integrated conceptual framework presenting each chapter logically and coherently. You may need to add linking text to establish the relationship between one chapter and the next.

*Cross-referencing:* A cross-reference is a note that contains information in another part of the thesis. It can be a core concept, idea, or method. It can happen between chapters or within a single chapter between sections. Using this skill, you can avoid unnecessary repetition and show the same idea from different points of view, the sample example in the other parts of the thesis, or a general concept applicable to specific facts. Another advantage is it allows you to present the material as a cohesive story as a whole because it sews through lines in your work from one idea in one chapter to another concept in a different branch. For instance, an original idea folds into other thought systems that came before it.

*Master's thesis:* A master's thesis should demonstrate that the candidate knows the relevant literature, principal discoveries, and theories and can produce significant scholarly work. The work should contain some original contributions.

*PhD thesis:* A PhD thesis must contain substantial contributions of new knowledge to the research field. It presents the results and original analysis, which should be significant enough to be published.

# CHAPTER 6

# Thesis Writing

**TOPIC OUTLINE**

Title page
Abstract
Acknowledgment
List of abbreviations
Chapter 1 Literature Review
Chapter 2 General Methodology
Chapter 3 to 6 Experimental Chapters
Chapter 7 General Discussion and Conclusion
Conclusion and significance
References
Appendix
Publications
Thesis template

## Title Page

The title page format is similar across institutions; however, you may want to check your institution's guidelines for specificities, including the margins, spacing, and font size. Usually, the title page has the thesis title, your name, the department and institution, the degree of the program (e.g., honors, master's, or PhD of Biomedical Science), and the submission date.

## Abstract

The abstract serves as a concise summary encapsulating the essence of your research. It should delineate (1) the research necessity, (2) your methodology, (3) your discoveries, and (4) their implications. Given that many, including potential employers, will primarily assess your expertise through your abstract, crafting a compelling narrative that effectively showcases your work and insights is vital. Typically, a thesis abstract spans between 250 to 500 words. It should comprehensively cover:

- Your specific research domain.
- Existing gaps in the research.
- Your central aim and objectives addressing the identified gaps.
- The methodology deployed for your objectives.
- Principal findings and results.
- The added value and relevance of your study to the broader field.

A poorly written abstract contains (1) too much background without defining the research area, (2) no explanation of the research gap and how to address it, (3) no definition of the research aims, (4) no mention of how you did the study, (5) no clear key findings, and (6) a bold claim of conclusion without supporting evidence.

Acronyms can hinder clarity in a presentation unless explicitly defined. It's advisable to minimize their use for clearer communication.

### Acknowledgments

You can include a section of *acknowledgments* giving gratitude and recognition to your supervisor, university, sponsor, funder, or anyone who supported you during your high-degree research study.

### Table of Contents

The *table of contents* is where you list the chapters and sections of your thesis alongside their page numbers. Usually, it should not have more than three pages. A table of contents can let the readers know your overall work at a glance and find the topic they want to know more about it.

### List of Abbreviations

A *list of abbreviations* is an alphabetical list of abbreviations and acronyms. An abbreviation is a shortened version of a term or phrase, e.g., μg for microgram. An acronym is a type of abbreviation constructed from the first letters of a term, e.g., BDNF for brain-derived neurotrophic factor or MI for myocardial infarction.

An abbreviation list in a thesis can improve readability and prevent continually looking for the definitions of abbreviations in the main text.

The first time you use an abbreviation or acronym, it is time to spell out the whole terminology or phrase followed by the abbreviation or acronym encased in parenthesis. After defining an abbreviation or acronym for the first time in your main text, you no longer need to use the entire term; instead, use the abbreviation.

For example, the literature suggests that brain-derived neurotrophic factor (BDNF) positively correlates with cognitive function measured in the young and adult population. However, those patients with severe depression, even young, have a low BDNF.

## Chapter 1 Literature Review

A thesis *literature review* requires a clearly defined topic as a starting point. First, you may provide a couple of leading sentences to set the context, explaining what is known and what is unknown within your field of research.

*Topic development:* A review of the topic development should provide a history, concept, or methodology that leads to the required studies. By doing this, the readers or reviewers may follow why your research is necessary.

*Keywords:* After you have decided on the research topic, the first is to define a list of keywords for the literature search. The keywords should be directly relevant to the concepts and variables of the research topic.

The structures can vary in presenting the research topic development.

- A chronological presentation emphasizes what has happened in the topic over time.
- A thematic-focused presentation addresses various aspects of the topic.
- A methodological approach describes the topic from different methods.
- A theoretical framework describes various theories, models, and definitions of the key concepts.

*Pivotal publications:* Find the critical publications with influential theories or findings that have changed the field's view or direction. The fundamental concept from these papers could indicate a future research direction.

*Research gap:* To define the research gaps or problems in knowledge bases. Build up the debates and justifications leading to the motivation of the proposed research.

A literature review should not just summarize the data. Instead, you should analyze, evaluate, and interpret data to provide a picture of the state of knowledge on the topic.

- The data summary provides an overview of the main points and then puts them together as a coherent story.
- Analyzing the data leans toward the quantitative effect, either increasing or decreasing, based on a summary analysis.
- Evaluating data leans toward qualitative, effective, ineffective, no effect, or strength or weakness.
- Interpretation provides the meaning after your analysis.
- The conclusion summarizes the key findings from your critical analysis.

- The significance describes the possible external validity.
- The research hypothesis and aim should be drawn, which are related to the research questions of your project.

## Chapter 2 General Methodology

The methodology of medical research varies from study to study. However, the chosen methods should be appropriate to address the research questions you set out to answer. The focus should be the plan of what you will do. The reviewer will evaluate the reliability and validity of your research.

*Reliability:* An unreliable or wrong methodology produces inconsistent or faulty results. The reader expects you to have followed accepted practices so that the conclusions you reach are valid.

*Repeatability:* The methodology needs to be repeatable, meaning anyone who uses the methods you write about should get the same conclusions you reached. It allows other researchers to undertake your study using the same design and compare their findings to yours. This is very important within academic research, as each study builds on previous studies.

### The research methodology of a thesis should include the following:

*Research design:* You need to demonstrate that you understand the research design theory and why you have chosen specific types of research design for your thesis. A high-degree study can be quantitative, quantitative, or mixed design; one control and one or multiple intervention group design; acute or chronic study design. A flawed research design or methodology would mean faulty outcomes.

*Measurements:* The measurements used in the thesis determine the outcomes. You should state what and why you have decided to observe or measure the specific parameters. The research questions should determine what to measure. In the thesis, you may want to state the research techniques, tools, and materials used.

*Data collection:* The data collection should match the aims and questions of your study. The research questions can be quantitative or qualitative, determining whether you need to collect qualitative or quantitative data. Usually, quantitative data collection is for experimental research, and qualitative information is for interviews and focused groups. Furthermore, observation studies, survey studies, secondary data collection, and archival research may require both quantitative and qualitative data collection.

*Data analysis:* Data analysis aims to understand, compile, process, and summarize the research data, from which you will find common response patterns. Then you can evaluate facts aiming to identify the rationale behind those outcomes. In addition, you may want to compare your discoveries with the information published in the literature.

*Statistical analysis:* Usually, the thesis methodology uses the last paragraph to describe the statistical analysis. This section explains the statistical tests used, the assumptions of these tests, the threshold score determined, the sample size desired, the experimental duration required, and the variables defined.

- T-tests analyze the differences between two groups and analysis of variance (ANOVA) for three or more groups.
- Regressions examine the impact of a variable on another variable.
- Correlation and chi-square tests examine the associations or relationships between variables.

## Chapter 3 - 6 Experimental Chapters

*Experimental chapters* are the central parts of a thesis. Usually, you have four empirical chapters for a PhD thesis, two or three chapters for a master's thesis, and one or two for an honors thesis.

*Overall:* The experimental chapters aim to tell the reviewers and readers the story that has emerged from your research findings. These chapters present the results, interpret the meaning, and raise discussions, arguments, and theories. These chapters explain all aspects of your original research. Therefore, it becomes essential to have careful thinking and planning before writing these chapters.

*Chapters:* Each experimental chapter could focus on one aspect of the story or be a standalone chapter. Therefore, it may independently contain the structure, including title, abstract, introduction, method, result, discussion, and conclusion. Preferably, each experimental chapter may be translated into a paper for publication.

In quantitative research, you may present the descriptive statistics first, followed by the results of each of the objectives investigated. The outcomes should be arranged to show how the data tests the research hypotheses and presented sequentially to respond to each research hypothesis.

*Presentation:* The experimental chapter presentation is not simply describing the data. In all cases, the presentation should have a logical organization that reflects (1) motivations to raise the research questions, (2) rationales for the research hypothesis, (3) statements of the research aim and objectives, (4) details of the research design, measurements, and analysis, (5) outcomes, and (6) discussions.

Rationales: As logical responses to the questions, hypothesis, aims, and even outcome interpretations, you need sufficient reasons to justify them. The data interpretation requires appropriate reasons for saying that data should be interpreted in one way rather than another. The explanations can be laid out by presenting one set of evidence that addresses your first question, followed by the next set of data that answers your second research question.

## Chapter 7 General Discussion and Conclusion

*Thesis story:* An overarching story of the thesis is a good starting point for the general discussion chapter. There is no need to start the literature review and rationales again. Instead, you could lay out all the results of your study. Organize them logically, draw connections between the findings, and then develop a coherent story for your thesis. It may focus on the interpretation and explain the meaning of your thesis study.

*Overarching:* Since each experimental chapter has already included the interpretation of specific findings, there is no need to repeat those. What you need to do is to interpret your findings as a whole. To produce an overarching and coherent story, you could lay out all findings and work out the stories across chapters. The key is that the highlights of the innovations should drive the interpretation. The approach can be to develop a couple of summary tables and figures. The number of tables and figures will depend on the results relevant to your research questions. The summary table collects the findings from all experimental studies. The table containing quantitative data will help you to write summary sections of quantitative analysis. The summary figure can help you write a qualitative analysis.

*To address the research hypothesis:* The general discussion provides an opportunity to show how your research results relate to the initial research hypothesis. For example, you could address the following questions:

- Does the research outcomes support the initial hypothesis? Why and how?
- Do the research findings support only part of the hypothesis? For example, you could explain why your study cannot answer the whole question.
- Do your results disagree with your hypothesis? If so, explain why and whether or not there are alternative interpretations.
- Did you find results outside of your initial hypothesis? Interpret the meaning of the findings and discuss why.

*Innovation paragraphs:* From the summary tables and figures, you should be able to identify the innovations that highlight your thesis study. The results from more than one chapter allow you to determine the innovation highlights, which is not the same idea you have already presented in the individual chapters. From the cross-chapter analysis, you should develop several highlight paragraphs. Accordingly, as a general discussion, here is the only place for you to outline the innovations or knowledge contributions combining the findings from different experimental chapters.

You could highlight and explain any new knowledge that your research contributes to the field of study. You may point out the agreements and disagreements between your data and that of others. The length of each innovation paragraph may contain about 250 words and try to avoid possible repetition.

*Paragraph structure:* Each section or paragraph may include a central idea supported by a summary of the findings, interpreted by literature review data and concluding the meaning. The research justifications do not belong here since this is a discussion chapter. However, if you want to include some reasons, keep it brief.

Here are some skills for you to write the innovation paragraph.

- *Summary:* The summary derived from several chapters can be for the entire thesis or a discussion paragraph. It needs to be brief on the main findings to address the ideas you originally proposed for investigations. The approach is to use your knowledge to synthesize the discoveries, leading to a coherent story.
- *Interpretation:* The interpretation is about explaining the meaning of your research findings, including the entire research project and individual discoveries. There are two key elements to incorporate into this discussion:

- Links between your research findings and hypotheses or questions.
- Links between yours and others: A successful discussion integrates your research with others', stating which research was done by others and which was done by you. Do they complement each other, or do they contradict each other?

- *Evaluation:* You may provide landing remarks or a point of taking home message at the end of each paragraph, including the conclusion, strengths, weaknesses, and significance.

*Avoid:* As a general discussion chapter, any background or justification should be brief to the minimum. You could provide an overarching rationale but not reintroduce the literature.

## Conclusion and Significance

This section should always refer to the statement of research questions, which direct you to define the contribution to the topic.

*Conclusion:* The conclusion summarizes the essential findings and emphasizes your field contributions. You should relate it to your original research aims, objectives, and hypotheses when writing. Therefore, make sure you have answered your initial questions.

*Significance:* The research significance aims to ensure readers and reviewers understand the impact of your work and how the thesis is unique; therefore, think about what is the critical research gap. A clear description of the study's implication and contribution also provides the reader with information about the research purpose. For example, what are the advancements or benefits derived from this study? You could describe general and specific contributions. In addition, you could indicate how your discovery contributes to part of the field's literature and how it will benefit future researchers.

*Recommendation:* Generally, researchers use their study conclusions to lead recommendations for future studies. For example, based on these conclusions, a prospective study could address the questions raised by this thesis study. In addition, further research may investigate the cause of or relationship between the risk factors and disease development to better understand these findings' implications.

## References

A *reference list* provides the details of all papers cited in the thesis. The listed articles, books, or book chapters should be cited in the text. Do not just list the documents without citation in the text. The format should follow the institution's guidelines for a high-degree research thesis.

## Appendix

A thesis can enclose appendices at the end. The *appendix* is where you can have extra data but not in the main body of the thesis.

- Supporting documents include raw data, questionnaires, materials, technical descriptions, and pilot studies.

- Declarations include statements from co-authors and permissions of copyright.
- Publications are collaborative between you and your colleagues during the study, and you can attach them in PDF format at the end of the thesis.

## Publications

High-degree research always has journal article publications before the end of your study. You can use these publications in your thesis if they belong to your degree study. In this case, the format can be a thesis by publication, publication embedded as chapters, or articles at the end as an appendix. You need to demonstrate a logical, coherent, or unified body of work by enclosing publications in your thesis.

As the first author, there should be no issue with claiming that you did most of the work and incorporating the paper as a chapter of your thesis. However, as a shared first authorship but not the first author, a clear justification must be made as to what extent you have contributed to the publication. Check it with your supervisor or check it against institution guidelines.

## Thesis Template

| |
|---|
| Title page |
| Abstract |
| Acknowledgments |
| Table of Contents |
| List of Abbreviations |
| Chapter 1 Literature Review |
| Chapter 2 General Methodology |
| Chapters 3 Experiment 1 |
| Chapter 4 Experiment 2 |
| Chapter 5 Experiment 3 |
| Chapter 6 Experiment 4 |
| Chapter 7 General Discussion, Conclusion, and Significance |
| References |
| Appendices |
| Publications |

PART FOUR

# Tables, Figures, and Writing Skills

CHAPTER 7

# Table

The *table* and *figure* allow the reader to understand data through visual content. A table provides for the presentation of details without becoming cumbersome in text. A high-quality figure attracts the reader's attention in presenting the critical findings and can help write the results and discussion section. Quality tables and figures are essential to writing and can increase the manuscript's chance of publication.

When do you need a table? When you have large amounts of data, present them in a table rather than in the text. There is no need to use a table if there are only a few data points. Since the text describes the primary findings and explains the results, the data with no significant difference and supporting data should be put in a table. Usually, there is no need to write all detailed calculations when you have too many data values. A table is a great way to present a large amount of quantitative data, exact values, and statistical analyses.

## Title

The *title* should describe what is presented in the table and be above the top row. A table should have a clear, descriptive title, which functions as the topic sentence of the table. It can be lengthy or short, depending on the discipline, but make sure that the title describes the data.

## Columns and Rows

The first column and top row are the variables and should be organized logically. The headings need to have units of measurement. Without units of measurement, the data cannot be interpreted correctly. In a research paper, elements are listed from top to bottom, with the comparisons made from left to right.

Usually, the first column presents independent variables. The reader's attention moves from the title to the variable headings sequentially. The variable headers should be as simple as possible and allow readers to quickly grasp what the table is about, for example, socio-demographics, clinical characteristics, laboratory measurements, and behavior data.

The top row has the subjects and their associated statistics.

## Body

The table *body* is where numerical or textual data is located. The content of a table can include the sample size, mean value, standard deviation or standard error of the mean, and statistical significance.

## Footnotes

A *footnote* explains the abbreviations and scientific terms included in the table, which assists readers in understanding the content. Abbreviations may be used in column and row headings and the data field. They must be defined according to the sequence in the table.

## Things to Avoid

*Blank cells:* You should avoid leaving blank cells in a table because this can mean data is unavailable, not detected, or detected but not detectable; the method is not applicable; or you have made a typo. In this case, you could use a symbol and define it in footnotes.

*Inconsistencies:* Data inconsistencies can exist between table, text, and figure, leading to questions on the reliability of the research. This could happen for many reasons; for example, the author did not update the final results in the table. Therefore, cross-checking all data throughout the paper is always necessary, e.g., abstract against the text and text against tables and figures.

*Repetitions:* You may avoid duplicating the same data presented in the text, table, and figure.

## A Clinical Study Table

Table 1: Sociodemographic and clinical characteristics of patient and healthy control groups

| Variables | Patient group (n=318) | Control group (n=310) | $X^2$ / t | *p* |
|---|---|---|---|---|
| Age, mean yr (SD) | 39.2 ± 13.1 | 38.5 ± 11.3 | 0.532 | 0.595[a] |
| Male, n (%) | 150 (42.7) | 74 (46.3) | 0.006 | 0.807[b] |
| WC (cm) | 87.5 ± 11.1 | 83.6 ± 8.9 | 3.844 | 0.001[b] |
| Overweight, n (%) | 145 (45.6 | 48 (30.0) | 10.75 | 0.001[a] |
| BMI (Kg/M$^2$) | 24.8 ± 3.3 | 23.3 ± 2.6 | 4.955 | 0.001[b] |
| Hyperglycemia, n (%) | 118 (37.1) | 37 (23.1) | 9.497 | 0.002[a] |

Footnotes: You can use footnotes to explain the abbreviations used in the table.

*Features:* The first column lists variables that depend on the title's topic. For example, this study investigates metabolic syndrome; therefore, the variables are related to metabolic syndrome parameters, e.g., WC: waist circumference, BMI: body mass index, and hyperglycemia. The top row has patient and control groups and statistical analysis. The patient and control groups allow comparison of the variables, followed by the last two columns, which are statistics. The superscript letter *a* ($^a$) means it was an independent t-test; superscript *b* ($^b$) was a chi-square test. Data is mean ± SD for continuous variables such as age, WC, and BMI, while % is used for categorical variables.

## A Repeated Measure Table

Table 2: Changes of metabolic parameters after n treatment.

| Parameter | baseline | 1st month | 6th month | 12th month |
|---|---|---|---|---|
| Weight (kg) | 106.85±17.69 | 91.60±19.46 | 90.38±18.72 | 82.25±19.14[a] |
| BMI ($kg/m^2$) | 38.34±5.69 | 32.20±4.92[a] | 29.42±3.80[a] | 26.71±3.57[a] |
| Waistline (cm) | 120.05±7.86 | 107.38±10.20[a] | 99.60±12.95[a] | 95±10.42[a] |
| LDL (mmol/L) | 3.39±0.91 | 3.27±0.87 | 2.94±0.46 | 3.36±0.50 |
| .... | | | | |

Footnotes: Statistical significant differences are indicated with superscript letters or symbols ($^{a, b}$) added after the test group, $p < 0.05$ vs. baseline.

*Features:* A repeated measure table can contain large amounts of data, as indicated in this table, from baseline to one, six, and twelve months of intervention. Statistical analysis uses $^{a}$ to show $p < 0.05$ or 0.01 compared with controls.

Also, you can use 95% confidence intervals to present the results to show the size and precision implications, away from the p-value as a chance for the results.

## A Review Table

Table 3: Review of literature data between high-fat intake and obesity.

| Study ID | Study sample | Study type | Laboratory measures | Study results | ...... |
|---|---|---|---|---|---|
| Paper 1 | | | | | |
| Paper 2 | | | | | |
| Paper 3 | | | | | |
| Paper 4 | | | | | |
| .... | | | | | |

Footnotes: To explain superscript or lower-case letters and symbols used in the table, such as $^{a, b, c}$, and *, #.

Features: A review table summarizes the data from the literature. (1) The first column is study ID, where you could have the first author and year of the paper. (2) The study sample is the human study case and the models for in vivo or in vitro studies. (3) Study type includes association or causal relationship. (4) Laboratory measurements are the parameters relevant to the study's topic. (5) Study results are the main findings of that study or summary points.

CHAPTER 8

# Figure

*Figures* are essential in academic publishing, including bar graphs, frequency histograms, scatterplots, drawings, maps, and photographs.

Writers must ensure that each figure they create serves a clear purpose. The content of the figure should align with the research design and the overarching objectives of the study. Mastering the art of designing impactful figures is crucial for reinforcing your paper's narrative. Every element within a figure should be intentional, whether highlighting differences, demonstrating associations, indicating causal effects, or narrating the essence of your research.

When using figures, you should always think of readers. What is the easiest figure for the reader to understand? How can you present the data most simply and effectively? Figures give a visual impact and deliver findings effectively; therefore, most readers prefer to look at figures and graphs rather than read lots of pages. However, if they are of poor quality, it discourages the reviewers or readers from continuing to read the full article.

## Figure Contents

Figures in academic work often encapsulate a primary idea, complemented by various sub-presentations like histograms, images, or line charts. It's uncommon these days to see a solitary histogram; instead, diverse representations combined to convey a single concept are the norm. Here are common types of figures:

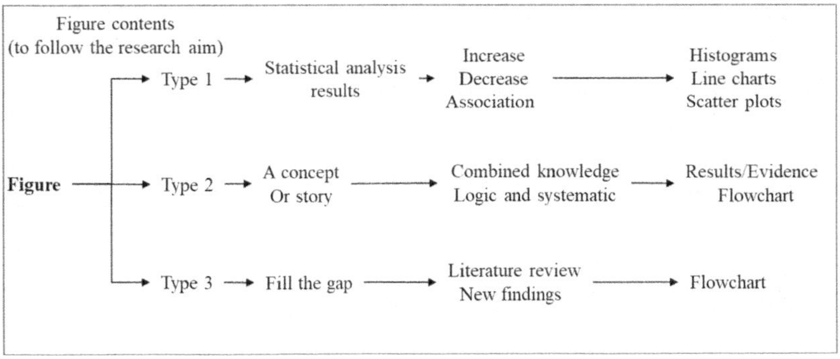


- **Type 1: Demonstrating Variations** - Such figures spotlight differences in study outcomes, be it an increase, a decline, or a static result. They might merge histograms, scatter plots, images, or line charts. It's advisable to maintain consistent measurements across similar categories.
- **Type 2: Conceptual Presentation** - Figures of this kind aim to elucidate an idea or narrative, underscoring a particular concept. Crafting these figures demands results from multiple experiments from varied angles to bolster the main idea. The outcomes from these diverse experiments should be sequenced logically and grounded in a solid scientific rationale, ensuring readers can grasp the concept's evolution seamlessly.

- **Type 3: Addressing Knowledge Gaps** - These figures shed light on areas where existing research might be scant. A flowchart proves effective here, first outlining the research theme and the existing knowledge void. Subsequently, it illustrates how the current research provides the missing insights.

Choosing the correct figures to represent data is a pivotal task that demands meticulous planning from the author. The nature of the data often dictates the most fitting type of figure. For instance, with continuous variables, one could consider:

1. Scatter Plot - To display individual data points.
2. Histogram - To provide a summarized view of data distributions.
3. Line Chart - Ideal for showcasing trends over time or variations with doses.
4. Bar Graph or Box Plot - Suitable for illustrating categorical variables.
5. Photograph - Beneficial when aiming to convey spatial relationships to readers."

## Figure Caption

The *figure captions* should be descriptive and easy to understand for readers; therefore, you should write the figure caption as accurately as possible.

Abbreviations and acronyms are helpful because figures always have space limitations. Figure captions should provide explanatory notes for the abbreviations and acronyms used in that figure.

You should include statistical tests, levels of significance, and even the sampling size used for analyses to facilitate an accurate understanding of the outcomes.

## Examples of figure captions

1. To summarize the meaning. UA improves fitness and extends lifespan (Ryu et al., 2016).
2. To describe the material. Chemical structures of EA and its derived metabolites UA, UB, UC, and UD (Ryu et al., 2016).
3. Results + intervention. The lifespan of worms treated with 50 μM EA, UA, UB, UC, or UD, or with vehicle (1% DMSO) (Ryu et al., 2016).
4. Results + Method. The lifespan of worms treated with 10, 30, or 50 μM UA, or the corresponding concentration of vehicle. (Ryu et al., 2016).
5. Results + time + intervention: Pharyngeal pumping at days 1, 7, and 14 of adulthood in worms treated with 50 μM UA or vehicle ($n = 10$)(Ryu et al., 2016).
6. Results + intervention + Methods. Effects of *in vitro*-positive mitophagy inducers on the induction of neuronal mitophagy in worms expressing mt-Rosella reporter (Xie et al., 2022).

## Histogram

A *histogram* shows the data using graphics in bars with different heights. Each bar depicts the outcome of statistical analysis with the means and standard deviation or standard error. The statistical differences are indicated with symbols indicating the *p*-values. It has independent variables on the horizontal axis and dependent variables on the vertical axis.

## Line Chart

A *line chart* is a graphical representation depicting information with data points connected by a line. It can display data that changes continuously over time. For example, a line chart can show the time effect, dose effect, or time-response curves.

A line chart can also be used in the method or result section and facilitate comprehension of the results obtained at specific steps of monitorization during the research process.

## Scatter Plot

A *scatter plot* uses dots to show the relationship between two different numeric variables. Usually, the independent variable is on the x-axis, and the dependent variable is on the y-axis. It can show either a positive, a negative, or no relationship between variables.

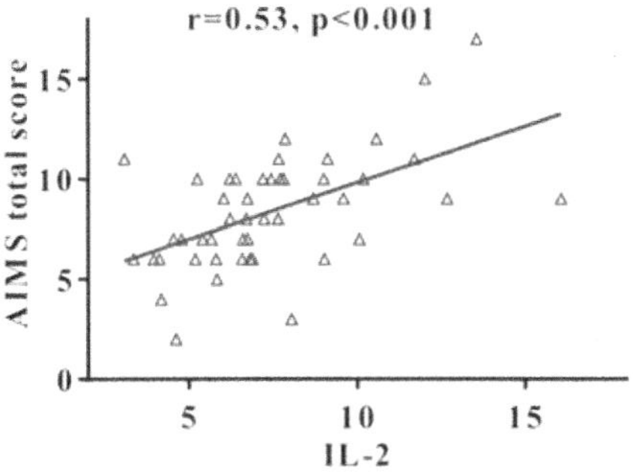


An example of a scatter plot to show the relationship between the plasma inflammatory cytokine IL-2 levels and abnormal involuntary movement scale (AIMS) scores in patients with tardive dyskinesia. There was a positive correlation between the levels of IL2 and AIMS total scores ($r = 0.53$, $p < 0.001$).

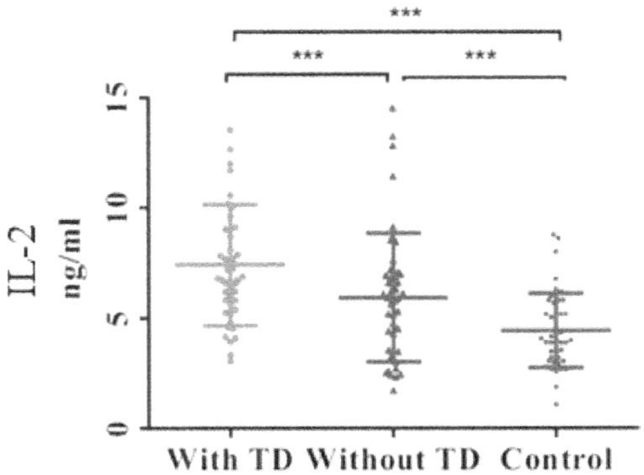


An example of a scatter plot shows the differences between the patients with and without tardive dyskinesia (TD), a movement disorder, and healthy controls (Control). *** $p < 0.001$

## Images

An *image* aims to have the writing visually attractive and easily understandable. You may consider the image's size, resolution, and visual attractiveness.

*Clinical image:* Medical images include an X-ray film, computerized tomography (CT), magnetic resonance imaging (MRI), ultrasound, and positron emission tomography (PET).

*Histological image:* Histological images aim to show the tissue microstructures. The gel images of protein and gene blots show the levels of a target protein and gene expression.

*Cell image:* Cell images show the morphology and content of the cells.

## Box Plot

A *box plot* presents group data in their quartiles. It can also show outlier data.

*Graphical abstract:* The PubMed website and some journals have begun to display thumbnails of figures or a graphical abstract alongside the paper's abstract. This is a visual summary of the main findings of the article.

CHAPTER 9

# Writing Skills

**TOPIC OUTLINE**

- Avoid poor logical flow
- How to write a paragraph
- Sentence construction
- Modifiers
- Agreement
- Word choice
- Precision

Logical flow in writing ensures a seamless and coherent progression of ideas, sentences, and paragraphs, minimizing ambiguity. In this context, "logic" refers to a structured and rational presentation of your narrative. Effective logical flow signifies the author's grasp on the intrinsic logic of the subject at hand. This entails leveraging sound reasoning and valid arguments to elucidate your ideas. Attaining clarity and precision in articulating the essence of research is paramount in scholarly writing. When ideas are presented logically, readers can effortlessly follow the narrative without getting sidetracked. Addressing and rectifying inconsistencies in one's writing can greatly enhance readability, allowing readers to grasp the core message both swiftly and intuitively.

**Example of Good Logical Flow:**

Dietary fiber intake has been widely recognized as an effective strategy for weight control among various age groups, especially older people. As people age, metabolism slows down, leading to potential weight gain and associated health risks. Incorporating fiber-rich foods, such as whole grains, fruits, and vegetables, into one's diet can promote feelings of fullness and reduce calorie intake. Additionally, dietary fibers improve gut health and boost metabolism, further assisting older adults in weight management. Thus, as the global population ages, there's an increased need for nutritional guidelines emphasizing the importance of fiber in senior diets.

**Example of Poor Logical Flow:**

Dietary fiber is good for older adults because it makes them feel full. Fruits, whole grains, and vegetables are foods that everyone loves. As we age, weight control becomes essential due to slower metabolism. The world is aging, so dietary guidelines are changing. Older people should consider fiber because it's beneficial for their gut health and overall weight control.

**Explanation:**

In the **Good Logical Flow** paragraph:

1. The primary topic, "dietary fiber intake for weight control among the elderly," is introduced clearly.
2. The paragraph then presents a logical progression of ideas: The challenge of a slowed metabolism in older age is

outlined, followed by dietary fiber's solution (satiety and reduced calorie intake). The broader implications for an aging global population and nutritional guidelines are also addressed.

3. Each sentence builds on the previous one, allowing the reader to follow a clear train of thought.

In the **Bad Logical Flow** paragraph:

1. Ideas are introduced randomly, making it challenging for the reader to follow the argument.
2. There's an abrupt mention of everyone loving certain foods, which doesn't directly relate to the importance of fiber and weight control for aged adults.
3. The world's aging and changing dietary guidelines are connected without a clear explanation or logical progression.
4. The sentences don't build on each other, causing the narrative to feel disjointed and confusing.

## Paragraph

Paragraphs serve as the foundational building blocks of a paper. Take, for instance, a scientific paper; it consists of distinct sections like the abstract, introduction, methods, results, and discussion. Each of these sections can be broken down into multiple paragraphs. It's essential for each paragraph to articulate a singular, central idea clearly and coherently, steering clear of diverging viewpoints.

**Opening Sentence:** This initial sentence sets the tone and introduces the primary theme or assertion. It creates a context for the subsequent details. One can approach this beginning with a:

1. **Rationale** - Highlighting prior research or existing knowledge (e.g., "Previous studies have indicated...," "Considering the prevalent evidence...")
2. **Objective** - Outlining the purpose or aim (e.g., "This study seeks to determine...," "Our objective was to elucidate...")
3. **Extension** - Proposing further inquiry based on existing data (e.g., "To delve deeper into this phenomenon...," "In light of these findings, we further investigated...")

**Supporting Sentences:** These sentences bolster the core idea introduced at the start. They furnish the paragraph with relevant evidence, detailed explanations, interpretations, and evaluative commentary.

**Concluding Sentence:** This final sentence encapsulates the presented data in relation to the central theme and establishes a segue into the subsequent paragraph. For instance, one might conclude with assertions like "The findings thus suggest..." or "Our results underscore..."

**Golden Rule:** Ensure that each paragraph is dedicated to elaborating on one specific idea, buttressed by relevant evidence and analysis.

**Example of a Good Paragraph:**

**Opening Sentence:** Previous studies have consistently underscored the significance of dietary fiber intake in weight management among overweight adults. **Supporting Sentences:** Dietary fibers, found abundantly in foods like whole grains, fruits, and vegetables, have been linked to heightened feelings of satiety and, consequently, reduced calorie consumption. This is primarily because fibers delay gastric emptying and increase food volume without adding calories, making individuals feel fuller for longer. Furthermore, fibers can modulate the gut microbiota, which plays an influential role in weight management and metabolic health. **Concluding Sentence:** Consequently, increasing dietary fiber intake emerges as a practical and sustainable strategy for weight control in overweight individuals.

**Example of a Poorly Written Paragraph:**

**Opening Sentence:** Dietary fiber is everywhere and overweight adults need it. **Supporting Sentences:** Some foods have a lot of fibers, like fruits and veggies. They help with feeling full, but they don't add to the calories. Fibers are good because they make your stomach take time to digest. There's also something about fibers and gut health. **Concluding Sentence:** So, eating more fibers seems to be a cool idea for people with weight issues.

**Explanation:**

In the **Good Paragraph**:

1. The **Opening Sentence** clearly references prior studies and introduces the central idea related to the significance of dietary fiber for weight control.
2. The **Supporting Sentences** elaborate on the mechanism by which fiber aids in weight control, providing specific examples and clearly linking cause and effect. The relationship between fiber and gut microbiota is also brought in as an additional layer of evidence.
3. The **Concluding Sentence** succinctly sums up the main idea and its implications.

In the **Poorly Written Paragraph**:

1. The **Opening Sentence** lacks specificity and sounds informal.

2. The **Supporting Sentences** are disjointed and lack a coherent flow. They are also simplistic and do not delve deeply into the topic.
3. The **Concluding Sentence** is casual in tone and fails to effectively encapsulate the main points.

The good paragraph offers a structured, detailed, and clear exposition of the topic, whereas the poorly written one is vague, lacks depth, and fails to maintain a professional tone.

**A Subtitle of a Paragraph:**

In research papers, the overall structure is crucial to ensuring clarity, coherence, and a logical progression of ideas. While the title provides a general overview of the paper's main theme or topic, subtitles (often referred to as subheadings) play a pivotal role in delineating specific sections or themes.

1. **Guidance for Presentation:** A well-chosen subtitle acts as a roadmap, directing the flow of information. When an author moves from one significant point or theme to another within a section, a subtitle signals this transition. This helps in organizing thoughts and ensuring that the narrative proceeds in a systematic manner.
2. **Relevance and Focus:** Subtitles ensure that the content presented beneath them stays relevant to that specific topic or theme. Authors are reminded to stick to the topic at hand by having a defined subheading, preventing unnecessary digressions. Readers also benefit, as they can immediately grasp the focus of the upcoming content and understand its relevance within the broader context of the paper.

3. **Improved Readability:** In dense or lengthy research papers, subtitles break down the content into digestible chunks. This segmentation allows readers to process information better, pause for comprehension, and even easily navigate to specific sections of interest.

4. **Enhancing Accessibility:** For readers who may be skimming the paper or are looking for specific information, subtitles act as signposts. They can quickly scan through the subtitles to locate the exact section or data they're interested in, making the paper more user-friendly.

In conclusion, subtitles are more than simple headings in a research paper. They provide structure, maintain focus, enhance readability, and improve the overall accessibility of the content. By employing effective subtitles, researchers can ensure their work is organized and easily understandable, allowing readers to engage more deeply with the presented findings.

**Example of Disjointed Paragraph**:

Dietary fiber can be found in many foods like fruits, vegetables, and whole grains. Overweight adults often struggle with their weight due to various factors. Intake of dietary fiber is linked with feelings of fullness. There's an obesity epidemic worldwide, and solutions are urgently needed. Feeling full can lead to less calorie consumption.

**Explanation**: The paragraph is fragmented in its approach to the topic. It jumps from introducing dietary fiber sources to discussing the challenges overweight adults face, then back to the benefits of dietary fiber, and finally to a broad statement about a global obesity epidemic. The connections between these statements are not clearly outlined, making it hard for readers to follow the logical progression of ideas.

**Improved Paragraph**: Overweight adults face an uphill battle in achieving weight maintenance, with the worldwide obesity epidemic highlighting the urgency of finding practical solutions. Dietary fiber, abundant in foods such as fruits, vegetables, and whole grains, plays a crucial role in this context. Dietary fiber promotes feelings of satiety, which can result in reduced calorie consumption, serving as a beneficial strategy for weight control among overweight individuals.

**Comments**: In the improved paragraph, the narrative starts by addressing the challenges overweight adults face, putting it into a broader context by mentioning the global obesity issue. Then, it transitions smoothly into the potential solution dietary fiber provides, detailing its benefits. This progression of ideas offers clarity and ensures that each point logically leads to the next.

## Construct Sentences

Sentences form the foundational blocks of any written piece. In constructing them, clarity and precision are paramount to prevent ambiguity. Each sentence should convey a distinct idea, ensuring a logical flow throughout the text. Scientific writing, in particular, prioritizes straightforward presentation. Thus, even those without expertise in the subject should find the sentences comprehensible. To achieve clarity, writers must employ concise, direct, and precise wording. Additionally, maintaining a consistent tone and style aids in producing text that flows seamlessly.

***Constructing a clear and simple sentence:***

1. **Focus on One Idea:** Ensure that each sentence expresses one clear point or idea.
2. **Use Active Voice:** Active voice makes it clear who is doing the action. For example, "The cat chased the mouse" is clearer than "The mouse was chased by the cat."
3. **Choose Simple Words:** Avoid jargon, complex vocabulary, or overly technical language unless necessary.
4. **Keep it Concise:** Eliminate unnecessary words. Instead of "In spite of the fact that," you can simply say, "Although."
5. **Be Specific:** Instead of saying "Some people prefer to...," say "Many adults prefer to..."

6. **Avoid Double Negatives:** They can be confusing. Instead of saying "I don't need no help," say "I don't need help."
7. **Structure Matters:** Use a subject-verb-object structure for clarity. For example, "She (subject) wrote (verb) the letter (object)."
8. **Stay Consistent:** Ensure that your sentence maintains consistent tense, voice, and point of view.

By adhering to these guidelines, your sentences will be more straightforward and easily understood by readers.

**Example of Clear Sentence**: "Dietary fiber intake can help prevent weight gain in elderly individuals." **Explanation**: This sentence is direct and to the point. It clearly states the relationship between dietary fiber intake and weight gain prevention in the elderly.

**Example of Non-Clear Sentence**: "When older people think about managing how much they weigh, the stuff they consume that's like roughage might play a part." **Explanation**: This sentence is wordy and uses vague terms like "stuff" and "like roughage" instead of directly stating "dietary fiber". The phrasing "think about managing how much they weigh" is also longer than simply saying "prevent weight gain". The overall structure makes the main point less evident to the reader.

***To keep the principle of avoiding redundancy:***

Example: A sentence should not have additional words that do not add other meanings. For example, A satiety control gene has been reported by several studies to be altered in obesity, and pathophysiological conditions based on genetic abnormality are being suspected (twenty-six words).

Revised: Avoid unnecessary words in a sentence. For instance, A satiety control gene reportedly influences obesity pathophysiology, prompting suspicions of genetic alterations (fifteen words). Eschew extraneous terms.

Example: In the majority of the experiments that were conducted over the span of two years, it was consistently found by the research teams that the application of this particular compound resulted in significant inhibition of the growth of cancerous cells in lab mice (thirty-six words).

Revised: Most two-year experiments showed that this compound significantly inhibited cancer cell growth in lab mice (fifteen words).

***Fragments:***

1. **Avoiding Truncated Meaning**:
    - Incorrect: "The drug, which was administered to the mice, who were in the experimental group, demonstrated effectiveness."
    - Improved: "The drug demonstrated effectiveness in the mice of the experimental group."

- Explanation: The first sentence has unnecessary clauses that make it long and convoluted. Streamlining the sentence brings clarity and directness.

2. **Combining Sentences with Contrasting Ideas**:
    - Original: "Our initial results indicated the presence of a particular protein. Later tests did not detect this protein."
    - Improved: "Our initial results indicated the presence of a particular protein; however, later tests did not detect this protein."
    - Explanation: Using transitional words like "however" allows for a smooth transition between contrasting ideas, making the context clear to the reader.

3. **Combining Sentences with the Same Ideas**:
    - Original: "The clinical trials were successful. As a result, the drug received FDA approval."
    - Improved: "The clinical trials were successful; therefore, the drug received FDA approval."
    - Explanation: "Therefore" provides a cause-and-effect connection between the two related ideas, merging them into one cohesive thought.

4. **Providing Rationales Using Parallel Sentences**:

   Example: "Patients receiving Treatment A showed improved mobility. Similarly, those on Treatment B demonstrated better pain management."

   Explanation: The parallel structure provides justification for the effectiveness of both treatments, highlighting their respective benefits in a comparative manner.

**Highlighting Content**:

- Original: "Based on our extensive research over a period of three years, examining various patient groups, and considering the diversity of genetic factors, we concluded that this new treatment regimen shows promise for a significant segment of the population suffering from the particular ailment."
- Improved: "After three years of research, we found that the new treatment is promising for many with the ailment."
- Explanation: The improved sentence is concise and to the point, which is essential when you want to emphasize or highlight key findings or statements in your research.

***Passive voice:***

The use of passive voice in biomedical research papers has long been a topic of debate. Historically, the passive voice was favored because it depersonalized the research, lending a sense of objectivity to the findings. However, many modern journals and researchers now prefer the active voice for its clarity and directness. That said, passive voice is not entirely obsolete, and its appropriateness may vary based on context.

**Here are some examples:**

1. **Avoiding Truncated Meaning**:
   - Passive: "The cells were treated with the drug, which was synthesized by our team."
   - Active: "Our team synthesized the drug and treated the cells with it."
   - Explanation: The passive sentence contains an unnecessary clause that could truncate the meaning. In the active version, the agent (our team) and action (synthesized) are immediately clear, providing a direct understanding of who did what.

2. **Combining Sentences with Contrasting Ideas**:
   - Passive: "A significant reduction was observed in Group A, but no change was seen in Group B."
   - Active: "Group A showed a significant reduction, but Group B remained unchanged."
   - Explanation: The active voice here provides a more direct contrast between the two groups, making it easier for the reader to grasp the differing outcomes.

3. **Combining Sentences with the Same Ideas**:
    - Passive: "The protein's presence was confirmed by Test A. Similarly, its abundance was noted by Test B."
    - Active: "Test A confirmed the protein's presence, and similarly, Test B noted its abundance."
    - Explanation: Using the active voice gives the agency directly to the tests, reducing ambiguity and making the connection between the two ideas more apparent.

4. **Providing Rationales Using Parallel Sentences**:
    - Passive: "Improved mobility was reported in patients receiving Treatment A. Enhanced pain management was observed in those given Treatment B."
    - Active: "Patients receiving Treatment A reported improved mobility. Similarly, those on Treatment B experienced enhanced pain management."
    - Explanation: The active voice establishes a direct connection between the treatment and its effects, making it easier for the reader to understand the causal relationship.

5. **Highlighting Content**:
    - Passive: "A promising outcome was observed from the new treatment regimen after rigorous testing."
    - Active: "After rigorous testing, we observed a promising outcome from the new treatment regimen."

- Explanation: Using the active voice emphasizes who did the observing and what was observed, making the main point clearer and more immediate.

In summary, while passive voice can sometimes be used effectively in biomedical research papers to depersonalize and objectify findings, the active voice often offers greater clarity, directness, and conciseness. Researchers should consider the context and the journal's guidelines when deciding on voice.

## Logical Flow in Articles

Clear and organized content is crucial for reader comprehension, especially in scientific articles. When an article lacks logical flow, it can become difficult to understand and detract from the main focus or objectives of the work.

**Causes of Disorganized Content:** Disorganization can manifest at various levels, from the overarching narrative down to individual sentences. Common indicators of a lack of logical flow include:

- Fragmented ideas that don't connect smoothly.
- Repetition of phrases or sentences.
- Incorporation of unrelated information or data without clear relevance.
- Inconsistencies in verb tenses.
- Misuse of words or terminology.
- Abruptly merging disparate ideas without adequate transition.

- Drawing conclusions without providing sufficient evidence or justification.

**Example of Good Logical Flow:** "Dietary fiber is essential for weight management in the elderly because it promotes a feeling of fullness and aids in digestion. As seniors often struggle with slowed metabolism and digestive issues, incorporating fiber-rich foods into their diets can be beneficial for maintaining a healthy weight."

**Example of Poor Logical Flow:** "Dietary fiber makes you feel full and is found in many vegetables. Elderly people often enjoy watching television during the evening."

The first example focuses on the topic and logically connects dietary fiber to weight management in older people. The second example begins on the issue but then introduces an unrelated idea about older adults watching television, disrupting the logical flow.

## Using Modifiers for Clarity in Research Citations

- **Differentiating Your Findings from Previous Work:** When discussing your research alongside other scholars', it's imperative to delineate clearly between your work and theirs. This differentiation ensures clarity and avoids misinterpretation by your readers.
- **Referring to Your Own Research:** To highlight your contributions, use direct, present-focused terms such as:

- "This research demonstrates..."
- "The findings of this study indicate..."

- **Citing Others' Research:** When referring to external works, it's best to provide specifics about the source:
  - "Huang et al. (2019) found that..."
  - "In a 2017 study conducted in Australia..."
- **Personalizing Your Contributions:** While maintaining objectivity, using the first person can also help emphasize your unique contribution:
  - "Based on my analyses, the data suggests..."
- **Drawing Comparisons with Previous Work:** To contextualize your work within the broader academic landscape, compare or contrast it with past findings or methodologies:
  - "Research from the 1980s echoed similar results, illustrating that..."
- These distinctions enhance the clarity of your writing and allow readers to trace the evolution of thought on the subject.

**Example of Good Use of Modifiers:** "In *this study*, we found that dietary fiber significantly aids weight management in elderly individuals, a finding that aligns with *Smith et al.'s 2020 research* on senior nutrition."

**Example of Poor Use of Modifiers:** "In the research, dietary fiber was found to be useful for elderly people. Some other people also studied this."

The first example clearly differentiates between the current study's findings and previous research by using precise modifiers ("this study" and "Smith et al.'s 2020 research"). The second example is vague, failing to specify which research or which "other people" are being referred to, leading to potential confusion for the reader.

### Understanding Dangling Modifiers

Dangling modifiers occur when a modifying phrase or word isn't clearly or logically related to the word it's intended to modify, often because the intended word is missing from the sentence. This can lead to confusion or unintentional humor.

Subjects can be either implied or explicitly stated. If implied, they often appear in the form of a phrase or clause. When a subject is explicitly stated, it needs to align with the verb, which, in turn, should correspond with the object.

To correct a dangling modifier, one must:

1. Identify the word the modifier is intended to describe.
2. Ensure that this word is present in the sentence.
3. Position the modifier so it directly precedes or follows the word it's meant to modify, ensuring clarity.

**Example of Dangling Modifier:** "*Hoping to garner benefits,* dietary fiber's consumption often increases in the elderly."

**Explanation & Improvement:** Here, the modifier "*Hoping to garner benefits*" seems to suggest that it's the "dietary fiber's consumption" that's hoping, which doesn't make sense. **Improved Sentence:** "*Hoping to garner benefits,* many elderly individuals often increase their consumption of dietary fiber."

**Example of Dangling Modifier:** "*After researching for years,* dietary fiber was found to be beneficial for weight management in the elderly." **Explanation & Improvement:** In this instance, "*After researching for years*" seems to suggest that the "dietary fiber" did the researching. This is not the intended meaning. **Improved Sentence:** "*After researching for years,* scientists found that dietary fiber is beneficial for weight management in the elderly."

In both examples, the problem arises when the modifier isn't placed next to the noun it's supposed to modify. By ensuring that the modifying phrase directly relates to the proper subject, the sentence becomes clearer and the modifier is no longer dangling.

### Distant Modifier

**Problematic Sentence with Distant Modifier:** "Elderly individuals often eat fruits high in dietary fiber with enthusiasm for weight management." In this sentence, the phrase "with enthusiasm" could be misinterpreted to suggest that it's the "dietary fiber" or "fruits" that have enthusiasm, which is illogical.

**Improved Sentence:** "Elderly individuals, with enthusiasm, often eat fruits high in dietary fiber for weight management." In the improved version, the phrase "with enthusiasm" is positioned closer to "Elderly individuals," making it clear that it's the individuals who are enthusiastic about eating fruits, not the dietary fiber or the fruits themselves.

**Problematic Sentence with Distant Modifier:** "People in their golden years often add dietary fiber to their meals for better digestion with a sense of urgency." Here, the phrase "with a sense of urgency" could be misinterpreted to suggest that it's the "digestion" or "dietary fiber" that has a sense of urgency, which is not the intended meaning.

**Improved Sentence:** "People in their golden years, with a sense of urgency, often add dietary fiber to their meals for better digestion." In this revision, the phrase "with a sense of urgency" is positioned closer to "People in their golden years," clarifying that it's the elderly individuals who are feeling the urgency to add dietary fiber for better digestion.

**Agreement in Writing**

1. **Subject-Verb Agreement**: The verb of a sentence should agree with the subject in number, whether singular or plural.

    - **Incorrect**: John and Lisa *discusses* science.

- **Correct**: John and Lisa *discuss* science.

Tip: Always ensure that the verb you choose matches the subject, singular or plural.

- **Incorrect**: The quality of the fruits *are* exceptional.
- **Correct**: The quality of the fruits *is* exceptional.

**Tip**: Collective nouns (like "quality" or "team") are often singular and need singular verbs.

- **Incorrect**: Neither the teacher nor the students *was* available.
- **Correct**: Neither the teacher nor the students *were* available.

**Tip**: When using "either...or" or "neither...nor", the verb should agree with the nearest subject.

2. **Noun-Pronoun Agreement**: Pronouns should agree in number (singular or plural) with the nouns they replace.

- **Incorrect**: Patients take *his* medication.
- **Correct**: Patients take *their* medication.

Tip: Be careful about generic pronouns, such as 'everyone' or 'anybody', which are often singular even though they sound plural.

- **Incorrect**: Each of the boys should bring *their* books.
- **Correct**: Each of the boys should bring *his* book.

**Tip**: Indefinite pronouns (like "each", "neither", "either") are typically singular.

- **Incorrect**: Neither of the women forgot *their* umbrella.
- **Correct**: Neither of the women forgot *her* umbrella.

**Tip**: Avoid making assumptions about gender unless specified. Use singular gender-neutral pronouns when applicable.

3. **Pronoun-Pronoun Agreement**: The pronouns in a sentence should maintain a consistent point of view.

- **Incorrect**: If *you* did not check the literature, *he* should not say based on the last ten years of research.
- **Correct**: If *you* did not check the literature, *you* should not say based on the last ten years of research.

Tip: Watch for shifts in pronoun perspective throughout a sentence or paragraph.

- **Incorrect**: If *one* wants to succeed in life, *you* have to work hard.
- **Correct**: If *one* wants to succeed in life, *one* has to work hard.

**Tip**: Maintain the same point of view throughout the sentence to avoid confusion.

- **Incorrect**: *We* should always stand by our friends, as *they* will stand by *you*.
- **Correct**: *We* should always stand by our friends, as *they* will stand by *us*.

**Tip**: Stay consistent with pronouns. Don't switch from plural to singular or vice versa.

4. **Verb-Verb Agreement**: The intention behind the verbs in a statement should be consistent. Using a verb that implies uncertainty followed by a definitive action can create confusion.

- **Incorrect**: Our results *suggest* that quinolinic acid *decreases* neural connectivity in multiple sclerosis.
- **Correct**: Our results *show* that quinolinic acid *decreases* neural connectivity in multiple sclerosis.

Tip: Ensure that the meaning behind the verbs you use in a sequence or in relation to one another is coherent.

- **Incorrect**: The research *indicates* that the drug *causes* an improvement, not cures it.
- **Correct**: The research *shows* that the drug *causes* an improvement, not cures it.

**Tip**: Ensure verbs maintain a consistent tone or level of certainty.

- **Incorrect**: The author *believes* that urban development *is* causing more harm than good.
- **Correct**: The author *argues* that urban development *is* causing more harm than good.

**Tip**: Ensure that verbs used in a sequence are logically and contextually related.

5. **Verb-Event Agreement**: The action described by the verb should logically match the event or situation it refers to.

- **Incorrect**: To evaluate the physiological role of a dopamine receptor, we applied eight doses of an antagonist on neurons, including 0, 10, 20, 40, 80, 160, 320, and 640 nM.
- **Correct**: To investigate the effects of various doses of an antagonist on neurons, we applied eight different concentrations, including 0, 10, 20, 40, 80, 160, 320, and 640 nM.

Tip: Make sure the action of your verb accurately describes the event or situation you are discussing.

- **Incorrect**: To understand the mechanics of the car, he drove to the countryside.
- **Correct**: To enjoy a leisurely drive, he went to the countryside.

**Tip**: Ensure the action or purpose stated at the beginning of a sentence aligns with the action or outcome presented at the end.

- **Incorrect**: To demonstrate the power of electricity, he wrote an essay.
- **Correct**: To highlight the importance of electricity, he wrote an essay.

**Tip**: Make sure the event or action specified by the verb accurately matches the context or scenario being presented.

By carefully observing these agreements, your writing will become clearer and more precise, ensuring effective communication of your ideas.

## Claim Certainty Levels

The levels of certainty you've presented can be helpful in understanding the degree of confidence one might have about a particular claim. They can be seen as a spectrum ranging from high certainty to more tentative knowledge. Here's a breakdown of each level:

1. **You are sure about the claim because you have reliable evidence for it.**
    - This suggests that there is solid, empirical evidence supporting the claim. For instance, scientific studies that have been peer-reviewed, widely accepted, and replicated could fall under this category. A claim like "smoking causes lung cancer" has a vast body of evidence supporting it, so one could be very sure about it.

2. **You are less certain about the claim because of incomplete evidence for it.**
    - This level acknowledges that while there might be some evidence for the claim, it's not comprehensive or conclusive. Such claims might be based on initial findings, anecdotal evidence, or data that has some limitations. For example, early research on a new medical treatment could indicate potential benefits, but more studies would be needed to confirm its efficacy and safety. In such cases, a degree of caution is appropriate when discussing or acting on the claim.

3. **You know it within certain realms of possibility.**
    - This level of certainty is even more tentative. It suggests that the claim is plausible based on what is currently known, but it's far from being proven. It could be based on theoretical considerations, educated guesses, or emerging patterns that haven't been rigorously tested. An example might be speculating about future technological advancements based on current trends. While it's possible they could occur, predicting the exact trajectory of technological development is challenging.

- It's essential to understand these levels when discussing claims or making decisions based on them. Knowing the level of certainty can help individuals avoid making overly confident decisions based on tentative evidence and help in evaluating the reliability of sources and information.

**Probability expressions from definite assertions to uncertainty:**

1. Smoking definitively causes lung cancer.
2. Smoking invariably increases the risk of lung cancer.
3. Smoking is proven to heighten the risk of lung cancer.
4. Smoking is very likely to cause lung cancer.
5. Smoking is likely to lead to lung cancer.
6. Smoking often results in lung cancer.

7. There is a good chance that smoking can cause lung cancer.
8. Smoking might cause lung cancer.
9. Smoking may potentially increase the risk of lung cancer.
10. Smoking could possibly lead to lung cancer.
11. There's a small chance that smoking relates to lung cancer.
12. Smoking is unlikely to cause lung cancer.
13. Smoking is rarely associated with lung cancer.
14. It's uncertain if smoking has any connection to lung cancer.
15. Smoking might or might not have any impact on lung cancer.

## Distance Yourself from the Definitive Claim

When distancing from a definitive claim, it's about softening the assertion, introducing ambiguity, or shifting the source of the claim to another entity. Here are some examples with explanations: Statement: Chocolate causes acne.

Distanced Versions:

1. Chocolate may cause acne.

Explanation: The word "may" introduces a possibility, not a certainty. It acknowledges that while chocolate might cause acne for some, it's not a guaranteed outcome for everyone.

2. Some studies indicate that chocolate can lead to acne.

Explanation: The claim is shifted to "some studies," which implies that not all research agrees with this statement. This also suggests that the claim isn't universally accepted and might only represent one perspective among many.

3. There's a belief that chocolate is linked to acne.

Explanation: By referencing "a belief," the statement introduces a level of societal or cultural hearsay without confirming the veracity of the claim.

4. It's been suggested that chocolate might be associated with acne.

Explanation: The phrase "it's been suggested" is non-specific about the source of the suggestion, thus removing direct responsibility from the statement. "Might be" adds an extra layer of uncertainty.

5. There's ongoing debate about chocolate's role in acne development.

Explanation: This highlights that the subject is still under discussion and lacks a definitive conclusion.

By distancing yourself from a definitive claim, you communicate a sense of uncertainty, acknowledge the existence of other perspectives, or emphasize that more information is needed before making a concrete statement. This can be useful in situations where evidence is inconclusive, where opinions are varied, or where it's important to avoid making sweeping generalizations.

### Make a Conservative Claim by Showing Its Limitations

When making conservative claims, it's helpful to highlight the limitations or specific conditions under which a claim holds true. This can be achieved by specifying the statement's scope, context, or boundaries. Here are the given sentences with explanations for how each one is conservative:

1. **According to a 2019 study, dietary fiber intake was beneficial for elderly participants with constipation.**

   **Explanation**: This claim is limited by both the date of the study ("2019") and the specific demographic ("elderly participants"). It doesn't generalize the benefit of dietary fiber for all age groups.

2. **While many individuals find relief from constipation with increased dietary fiber, it's not effective for everyone.**

**Explanation**: The qualifier "many" acknowledges a general trend but also makes clear that there are exceptions by stating "it's not effective for everyone."

3. **In a controlled setting, subjects who consumed more dietary fiber reported fewer instances of constipation.**

**Explanation**: The phrase "in a controlled setting" suggests that the study was conducted under specific conditions that might not necessarily reflect real-world situations for everyone.

4. **Soluble fiber, found in oats and beans, has been linked to improved bowel movements in some populations.**

**Explanation**: The specification of "soluble fiber" and the examples give a more narrowed focus. Additionally, "some populations" indicates that the benefit isn't universal across all demographics or groups.

5. **Dietary fiber can alleviate constipation, but its efficacy can vary based on the individual's overall diet and hydration level.**

**Explanation**: This claim recognizes the potential benefits of dietary fiber but also introduces other variables ("overall diet and hydration level") that can influence its effectiveness.

By introducing specifics like study dates, demographics, conditions, or types of fiber, these claims avoid making sweeping generalizations and instead present a nuanced view that acknowledges the complexities of the topic.

## Drawing conclusions and discussing the implications of research findings

1. **Implication to Current Knowledge and Theory**:

   Every new research study should ideally contribute to the existing body of knowledge. This may involve either supporting or refuting current theories or even proposing new ones.

   For example, if a study finds a new mechanism by which a particular protein affects cell growth, but the study was conducted only in vitro (outside a living organism), a limitation could be that the findings might not exactly translate to in vivo (within a living organism) situations.

2. **Technical Applications or Clinical Practice**:

   If your research can be directly applied to a practical scenario, it is essential to outline how it might be used in the real world. This has huge implications, especially in fields like medicine where new research can change clinical practices.

For instance, if a new imaging technique might be effective in detecting tumors in early stages under controlled lab conditions. However, a limitation might be that in a real clinical setting with various patient demographics, the tool's efficacy might vary.

3. **Discussion and Conclusion**:
   - **Interpretation of the results**:
     - **Example**: If the sample size of a drug trial is small, the conclusion might not be generalizable to a broader population.
   - **Significance of the work**:
     - **Example**: A study may find a statistically significant reduction in blood pressure with a new medication, but the actual reduction might be clinically insignificant, say, a reduction of only 1-2 mmHg.
   - **Application of outcomes**:
     - **Example**: A drug might be effective in a controlled research environment, but its efficacy may differ when other real-world variables come into play, like patient adherence to medication or interactions with other medications.

4. **Distinguishing New Findings**:
   - A study might reveal that a particular gene mutation is more common in patients with a specific disease.

However, the limitation could be that the population studied was from a specific geographical region, making it uncertain if this mutation-disease association holds true in other populations.

5. **Careful Wording**:
    - As researchers, it's crucial to be precise and avoid over-generalization. Phrases like "may contribute to," "suggests," or "is associated with" are often more accurate than definitive claims unless the evidence is overwhelmingly conclusive.
    - Overstatements or oversimplifications can mislead readers, so always ensure that claims made are backed by the evidence presented in the research.
    - **Example**: If a study suggests that a particular diet is linked with reduced risk of a certain disease, but the research is based on self-reported food diaries, a limitation would be the accuracy and honesty of self-reporting by participants.

6. **Avoiding Definitive or Strong Claims**:
    - The example you provided about dietary fiber and cardiovascular disease is a good one. Instead of a blanket statement, it would be more accurate to say something like "increased dietary fiber intake has been associated with a reduced risk of cardiovascular disease in certain populations."

- Using qualifiers allows for the fact that research often has limitations, such as a specific sample size, demographic, or methodology.
- **Example**: A research finding might suggest that stem cell treatment helps in improving heart function post a cardiac event. However, if this study was done only on animals and not humans, a limitation is the potential differences in response between species.

It's essential for researchers to transparently convey these limitations. This not only builds trust but also provides direction for future studies to address and overcome these constraints.

## Words

### Unnecessary Words

Using more words than needed (often termed "wordiness") can obscure the message and make writing harder to read. Clear and concise writing helps convey information efficiently.

1. **Be Direct**: Avoid beating around the bush. Get to the point.
    - Wordy: Researchers have undertaken a study, and the results from this study seem to suggest that a specific gene may play a role in the progression of colon cancer.
    - Concise: A recent study indicates a specific gene's role in colon cancer progression.

- Wordy: Due to the fact that it was raining, he decided he would not go to the park.
- Concise: Because it was raining, he didn't go to the park.

2. **Use Active Voice**:

   Instead of "The game was watched by Mary," use "Mary watched the game."

   - Passive: The association between dietary fiber intake and colon cancer risk was studied by our team.
   - Active: Our team studied the association between dietary fiber intake and colon cancer risk.

3. **Remove Redundant Words and Phrases**:

   Phrases like "completely finished" or "true facts" have redundant words.

   - Redundant: Our preliminary results are in fact showing a positive correlation between red meat consumption and colon cancer risk.
   - Concise: Our preliminary results show a positive correlation between red meat consumption and colon cancer risk.

4. **Avoid Fillers**:

   Words and phrases like "actually," "basically," and "in order to" often don't add meaning.

- Wordy: Basically, in order to understand the disease's genetic factors, we analyzed DNA samples from colon cancer patients.
- Concise: We analyzed DNA samples from colon cancer patients to understand the disease's genetic factors.

5. **Revise and Proofread**:

   After writing, go back and review your work to see if there are words or sentences that can be refined.

- Before Revision: We conducted a research study where we decided to use a cohort of 1,000 patients to see if there might be any sort of potential link between colon cancer and sedentary lifestyles, a topic that hasn't been deeply studied yet.
- After Revision: We studied a cohort of 1,000 patients to explore the potential link between colon cancer and sedentary lifestyles, an under-researched topic.

Applying these principles consistently in scientific writing helps ensure that the research is communicated effectively and can be more readily understood by peers, policymakers, and the public.

## Modifying Words

The use of certain modifying words can sometimes dilute or confuse the primary message of a sentence. They may be used for emphasis or to sound more authoritative, but they can also detract from clarity.

1. **Very**:

   Original: "A high-fat diet is very detrimental to metabolic health."

   Revised: "A high-fat diet is harmful to metabolic health."

2. **Basically**: This term often serves as filler and can usually be removed without altering the meaning of a sentence.

   Original: "High-fat diets basically lead to weight gain and increased risk for diabetes."

   Revised: "High-fat diets lead to weight gain and an increased risk for diabetes."

3. **Generally**:

   Original: "Mice that are fed a high-fat diet generally become obese."

   Revised: If you're acknowledging exceptions: "Most mice fed a high-fat diet become obese."

   If you're making a general statement: "Mice fed a high-fat diet become obese."

4. **Specifically**: This should be used when highlighting a particular aspect of a broader topic. If it's not narrowing focus, it might not be necessary. As in your example, "specifically" is extraneous.

5. **Precisely**:

   Original: "Mice on a high-fat diet gained precisely 20% more weight than those on a standard diet."

   Revised: If you're emphasizing the exactness of the measure: "Mice on a high-fat diet gained exactly 20% more weight than those on a standard diet."

   If exactness isn't the focus: "Mice on a high-fat diet gained more weight than those on a standard diet."

To maintain clarity in writing or speaking, it's always a good idea to:

- **Re-read sentences** without the modifier to see if the primary message remains unchanged.
- **Avoid filler words** that don't contribute to the message.
- **Be direct and succinct**. Brevity can often lead to clearer communication.

## Selecting a Meaningful Verb

In biomedical research, the choice of verbs is crucial, as it can convey the degree of confidence, causation, or correlation. Here are several examples with explanations:

1. **Tends to lower**:
   - **Example**: Regular exercise tends to lower the risk of heart disease.
   - **Explanation**: This statement implies that people who exercise regularly often experience a reduced risk of heart disease, but it's not a guaranteed outcome for everyone. In other words, while exercise often leads to better heart health, there may be exceptions.

2. **Contributes to reducing**:
   - **Example**: Regular exercise contributes to reducing the chances of developing heart problems.
   - **Explanation**: Here, the emphasis is on exercise being one of many potential factors that can help reduce heart problems. It implies that exercise plays a part in the overall picture of heart health, but other contributing factors could be diet, genetics, or stress management.

3. **Contributes to lowering**:
   - **Example**: Most research suggests that hitting the gym regularly contributes to lowering one's chances of facing cardiovascular issues.

- **Explanation**: Like the previous example, this structure emphasizes that regular gym workouts play a role in improving cardiovascular health. The use of "lowering" specifically describes the action that's taken on the chances of facing heart-related issues.

4. **Demonstrates vs. Suggests**:
   - **Example**: The study **demonstrates** a direct link between smoking and lung cancer. The study **suggests** a potential link between artificial sweeteners and weight gain.
   - **Explanation**: "Demonstrates" implies a stronger, more definitive finding. When a study demonstrates something, it means the evidence is compelling. On the other hand, "suggests" indicates a more tentative conclusion, possibly requiring more research for validation.

5. **Indicates vs. Speculates**:
   - **Example**: Bloodwork **indicates** elevated cholesterol levels in patients on this medication.
   - The paper **speculates** that these drugs might influence gut bacteria.
   - **Explanation**: "Indicates" implies there's data or tangible evidence pointing to a specific conclusion. "Speculates" suggests that there's a hypothesis or theory without solid evidence yet.

6. **Supports vs. Refutes**:
    - **Example**: The evidence **supports** the idea that omega-3 fatty acids benefit heart health. Recent research **refutes** the claim that vitamin C can cure the common cold.
    - **Explanation**: "Supports" conveys that the evidence aligns with and upholds a particular hypothesis or belief. In contrast, "refutes" means that the evidence contradicts or debunks a previously held idea.

7. **Correlates with vs. Causes**:
    - **Example**: High sugar intake **correlates with** an increased risk of Type 2 diabetes. The virus **causes** severe respiratory distress in certain individuals.
    - **Explanation**: "Correlates with" implies a relationship between two variables but doesn't necessarily mean one leads to the other. "Causes" indicates a direct effect where one variable produces an outcome in another.

8. **Enhances vs. Mitigates**:
    - **Example**: This drug **enhances** cognitive function in Alzheimer's patients. The treatment **mitigates** the side effects of chemotherapy.
    - **Explanation**: "Enhances" implies an improvement or elevation in the condition or state of something. "Mitigates" suggests that something reduces or alleviates adverse effects or situations.

The choice of verbs in biomedical research is crucial because it directly affects how findings are interpreted. A statement's strength, direction, and certainty can change substantially based on verb selection.

# CHAPTER 10

# Tense

**TOPIC OUTLINE**

Present simple tense
Past simple tense
Present perfect tense
Mixed tense
Tenses in the paper structure

Tense is commonly described as a "verb-based" approach to indicating the timing of an event. The most frequently used tenses in scientific paper writing are the present simple, past simple, and present perfect. These tenses can be applied in both passive and active voices.

Generally, reporting facts necessitates the use of the present simple tense, concepts that remain relevant to the present are expressed in the present perfect tense, and specific past events or actions are described using the past simple tense.

| | Present | Past | Future |
|---|---|---|---|
| *Simple* | I do it everyday.<br>s + v1+ O | I did it yesterday.<br>s + v2 + O | I will do it tomorrow.<br>s + 'will' + v + o |
| *Continuous* | I am doing it right now<br>s + 'am/are' + (v + ing) + o | I was doing it when you arrived.<br>s + 'was/were'+ (v + ing) + o | I will be doing it when you arrive.<br>s + 'will be' + (v + ing) + o |
| *Perfect* | I have done all jobs.<br>s + 'have/has' + v3 + o | I had done all job when you arrived.<br>s + 'had'+ v3 + o | I will have done all jobs by the time you arrive.<br>s + 'will have' + v3 + o |
| *Perfect continuous* | I have been doing it for 2 hours.<br>s + 'have/has' + (v + ing) + o | I had been doing it for 2 hours when you arrived.<br>s + 'had been' + (v + ing) + o | I will have been doing it for 2 hours when you arrive.<br>s + 'will have been' + (v + ing) + o |

Abbreviations: s, subject; o, object; v: verb (v1: present, v2: past, or v3: past participle)

## Present Simple Tense

The present simple tense is the first choice unless there is a reason for other tenses in a research paper. The present simple tense is versatile and plays a significant role in academic writing, especially in research papers. The clarity it brings to sentences makes it ideal for representing consistent and established facts. Here's a breakdown of the examples you provided and the roles the present simple tense plays in each:

1. **General statement:** This sets the stage by providing context. It's an overview or introduction to the topic or subject of the research. The present simple tense here conveys facts or established knowledge about the topic.

   **Example:** "Heart disease remains a leading cause of mortality worldwide."

   **Explanation:** The present simple tense in "remains" suggests a consistent, ongoing reality about heart disease, emphasizing its significance and relevance.

2. **Main aim:** Clearly state the purpose or objective of the paper. The use of the present simple tense underscores the ongoing relevance of the research.

   **Example:** "This study investigates the correlation between exercise frequency and mental well-being."

   **Explanation:** The verb "investigates" indicates the ongoing and present relevance of the study's purpose.

3. **Known topic:** Reinforce previously established facts or concepts. This is especially useful in the introduction or conclusion sections of a paper, where one might be summarizing what is known about a topic.

   **Example:** "Vitamin C plays a crucial role in boosting the immune system."

   **Explanation:** "Plays" in the present simple tense reiterates a well-acknowledged fact about Vitamin C, making the statement sound grounded.

4. **Citation without author's name:** This provides supporting evidence from other research. The use of present simple when citing sources suggests the enduring validity of the cited research.

   **Example:** "Honey possesses antibacterial properties (Smith, 2018)."

   **Explanation:** The verb "possesses" asserts the enduring trait of honey, which remains true regardless of when the cited research was conducted.

5. **Tables and figures:** Refers to visual data representations in the paper. The use of the present simple tense here emphasizes the immediate availability and relevance of the data.

   **Example:** "Figure 3 displays the annual sales of the company over the past decade."

   **Explanation:** The verb "displays" in the present simple indicates that anyone reviewing the research can refer to Figure 3 for that specific data at any point.

6. **Interpretations:** Here, the researcher interprets the data or findings. The present simple tense is used to convey the ongoing significance or relevance of the interpretation.

   **Example:** "The data indicates a significant increase in sales after implementing the new marketing strategy."

   **Explanation:** The use of "indicates" allows for a direct, real-time observation and interpretation of the findings.

7. **Discussion:** The present simple tense helps draw conclusions or extrapolate implications from the research findings. Stating these in the present tense underscores the current relevance of these conclusions or implications. **Example:** "The findings suggest that shorter sleep duration correlates with higher stress levels."

   **Explanation:** "Suggest" in the present simple highlights the paper's current understanding and interpretation of the results.

8. **Conclusion:** Here, the research is summarized, and the overarching findings are presented. The present simple tense solidifies the findings, making them sound well-established and relevant.

   **Example:** "The experiment confirms that light intensity affects plant growth rates. The increased light leads to accelerated growth."

   **Explanation:** "Confirms" and "leads" in the present simple tense underline the present and continuing implications of the research findings.

Using the present simple tense in these contexts provides *clarity* and emphasizes the ongoing relevance of the statements made. It also aids in making the research sound objective and grounded in evidence.

## Past Simple Tense

In biomedical research papers, the past simple tense is often used to describe specific actions, observations, or findings that took place at a definite time in the past. Here are some common scenarios where past simple tense is used:

1. **Methodology**: This section details what was done in the study.

   **Example**: We injected the mice with 10mg/kg of the drug daily for a week.

**Explanation**: This sentence describes a specific action (injection) that was done in the past over a set period of time.

2. **Results**: Here, researchers report on their specific findings.

   **Example**: The treated group exhibited a significant decrease in inflammatory markers compared to the control group.

   **Explanation**: The results of the observation are stated as a fact, indicating what was found in the past when the experiment was conducted.

3. **Previous Research**: Researchers often refer to previous findings to contextualize their study.

   **Example**: Smith et al. (2019) demonstrated that the XYZ protein played a pivotal role in cellular apoptosis.

   **Explanation**: Here, a past study is cited to indicate what was previously found or established.

4. **Data Analysis**: Details about how the data was interpreted.

   **Example**: Statistical analysis revealed a p-value of less than 0.05, indicating a significant difference.

   **Explanation**: The data was analyzed (in the past) and this is the result that was found.

5. **Observations**: Specific observations made during the course of the research.

   **Example**: Under electron microscopy, the cellular mitochondria appeared fragmented.

   **Explanation**: A specific observation was made using electron microscopy in the past, hence the use of past tense.

6. **Events in the Study**: Specific events or circumstances that happened during the research.

   **Example**: During the second phase of the trial, two participants experienced severe allergic reactions.

   **Explanation**: This sentence reports an event that occurred during the trial, indicating a past event.

Using the past simple tense in these contexts provides clarity and avoids ambiguity about the timing of events or observations. Readers can clearly understand that the actions or observations took place in the past, which is crucial for the credibility and replicability of scientific studies.

## Present Perfect Tense

In biomedical research papers, the present perfect tense is employed for a number of reasons, reflecting the unique considerations of scientific writing. Here are some common uses and examples:

1. **Recent or Relevant Findings:**

***Explanation:*** When researchers want to emphasize recent findings that have relevance or importance to the current study, they might use the present perfect.

***Example:*** "Scientists have recently identified a new strain of the virus that is resistant to traditional treatments."

Here, the implication is that the identification is recent and has significance in the current context.

2. **Past Research with Present Relevance:**

   ***Explanation:*** This usage emphasizes past research findings that still hold relevance in the current study context.

   ***Example:*** "Researchers have consistently found a significant association between smoking and lung cancer."

   The past studies are still relevant and important for the current discussion.

3. **General Trend or Consensus:**

   ***Explanation:*** The present perfect can indicate a repeated action or established understanding over time.

   ***Example:*** "Various studies have confirmed the role of oxidative stress in neurodegenerative diseases."

   The confirmation has taken place over various studies and still stands.

4. **Emphasizing Continuity:**

***Explanation:*** If there's an ongoing trend or phenomenon, which began in the past and continues to be valid now, the present perfect is used.

***Example:*** "The global community has been increasingly focused on potential therapies for Alzheimer's disease over the past two decades."

The focus started in the past but is still ongoing.

5. **Reporting Negative Findings:**

   ***Explanation:*** Sometimes, it's important to emphasize what hasn't been done or discovered in prior research to illustrate the novelty or gap the current research addresses.

   ***Example:*** "To date, no study has conclusively proven the efficacy of drug Z in treating this condition."

   This emphasizes the absence of such a study until now, potentially leading to the current study's importance.

6. **Setting the Stage for New Research:**

   ***Explanation:*** By acknowledging what has been understood or done up to the current point, authors can pave the way for their novel findings or methodologies.

   ***Example:*** "While several teams have explored the genetic basis of the disorder, the exact genes involved remain undetermined."

The implication is that while past research has been conducted, there's still room for discovery, which the current paper might address.

Understanding these nuances in tense usage can help readers better appreciate the context and significance of statements made in biomedical research papers.

## Mixed Tenses

Mixed tenses are often used in biomedical research papers to delineate between previously established knowledge, methodologies employed, and new findings or interpretations. Here are more contextual examples specifically from the biomedical research domain, along with explanations:

1. **Background Information vs. Current Study**
    - **Example**: "Several studies have demonstrated that BRCA1 mutations increase breast cancer risk, but our current analysis indicates a potential protective role in ovarian cancer."
    - **Explanation**: The past tense ("have demonstrated") references prior work, whereas the present tense ("indicates") pertains to the present study's findings.

2. **Time Shift (using past and present simples)**

- **Example**: "In 1995, John postulated that an obese subject has high cholesterol in circulation."
- **Explanation**: The sentence has a shift in time. "In 1995" indicates a specific past event, hence "postulated" is in the past simple. The statement of the hypothesis "an obese subject has high cholesterol" is presented in present simple to express a general fact or theory.

3. **Previous Findings vs. Current Interpretation**
   - **Example**: "Jones et al. (2015) reported higher levels of the neurotransmitter serotonin in depressed patients; however, our data suggest that its metabolite, 5-HIAA, might be the more relevant marker."
   - **Explanation**: Past research results are presented in past tense ("reported"), but the interpretation or findings of the current research are in the present tense ("suggest").

4. **Method Description vs. Study Outcome**
   - **Example**: "We utilized fluorescence microscopy to observe cellular structures, and detected significant morphological changes post-treatment."
   - **Explanation**: Methodology is presented in the past tense ("utilized"), indicating actions completed during the study, while findings from those methods are also presented in past tense ("detected"), showing what was discovered.

5. **General Truth vs. Specific Study Result**

    - **Example**: "Insulin typically regulates glucose uptake in cells, but our observations reveal an alternative pathway in insulin-resistant subjects."
    - **Explanation**: A general fact is stated in the present tense ("regulates"), whereas the new findings are in the present tense as they relate to the current study ("reveal").

6. **General Statement vs. Specific Findings (using present and past simples)**

    - **Example**: "Our results support the hypothesis that a high-fat diet increases body weight."
    - **Explanation**: "Our results support" is in the present tense, indicating the conclusions derived from the current study. "A high-fat diet increases body weight" is a general statement, hence it's presented in the present simple.

7. **Study Aim vs. Result**

    - **Example**: "We sought to identify novel biomarkers in Alzheimer's disease and discovered a potential role for protein Z."
    - **Explanation**: The study's intention is shared in the past tense ("sought"), and the outcome of that intention is also conveyed in the past tense ("discovered").

8. **General Claim vs. Specific Past Research**
    - **Example**: "The most commonly discussed phenomenon in music cognition is the Mozart Effect." followed by "Rauscher and colleagues first documented this effect in their seminal paper."
    - **Explanation**: The first sentence provides a general claim about the popularity of a phenomenon and uses present simple. The second sentence cites a specific study, so "documented" is in the past simple to reflect that this was an event that occurred in the past.

9. **Describing Figure or Table in Present vs. Past Data Collection**
    - **Example**: "Table 2 displays the patient demographics, which were collected between 2015 and 2020."
    - **Explanation**: The present tense ("displays") describes the current status of the table, whereas the past tense ("were collected") refers to the time when the data was gathered.

10. **Literature Observation vs. Implication of Current Study**
    - **Example**: "Past research linked gene X to obesity, yet our findings implicate an upstream regulator as the primary driver."
    - **Explanation**: Previous studies are referred to in the past tense ("linked"), while the current study's

conclusions are given in the present tense ("implicate").

11. **From Fact to Concept (using present vs. present perfect)**
    - **Example**: "Increased cytokine levels play a role in neurodegeneration." followed by "Neurodegeneration has been shown to be associated with increased cytokines."
    - **Explanation**: The first sentence presents a general fact in the present tense. The second statement uses the present perfect "has been shown" to express the idea that this is an established concept derived from previous research or observations.

Using tenses appropriately in biomedical research papers ensures clarity and helps convey the timeline and significance of the presented research in relation to the broader scientific knowledge.

## Tenses in the Paper Structure

The proper tense helps the reader understand the sequence of events, differentiates between established facts and the study's findings, and ensures clarity. Here's a breakdown of how tenses are typically used in the various sections of a biomedical research paper:

1. **Title**:
    - Typically present tense, but depends on the specific focus of the research.
    - Example: "The Effect of Drug X on Blood Pressure in Adult Patients."

      Present tense used to give a straightforward, general statement about the content of the study

2. **Abstract**:
    - **Background or Objective**: Present tense for general statements or established facts.
    - **Methods and Results**: Past tense when describing what was done and found in the study.
    - **Conclusions**: Present tense to summarize the implications of the findings.
    - Example: "Hypertension is a common condition. We studied the impact of Drug X on blood pressure in 200 adult patients. Patients administered with Drug X showed a significant reduction in blood pressure."

Present tense ("is") for established facts.

Past tense ("studied", "showed") for specific actions or findings from the study.

3. **Introduction**:
   - **Background information**: Present tense for established facts and generally accepted knowledge.
   - **Purpose or rationale of the study**: Present tense when stating the aim or goals.

     Example: "Hypertension affects millions worldwide. This study aims to explore the efficacy of Drug X in treating hypertension."

     Present tense ("affects", "aims") for ongoing situations and stating the study's purpose.

4. **Methods**:
   - **Procedure**: Past tense, as this section explains what the researchers did.
   - **Equipment or materials**: Present tense when describing the properties or characteristics of tools or materials.

     Example: "We administered Drug X to 100 patients, while 100 received a placebo. Blood pressure was measured using a standard sphygmomanometer."

Past tense ("administered", "received") for actions performed.

5. **Results**:
    - Past tense exclusively, since this section discusses specific findings and observations made during the study.

      Example: "Patients who received Drug X exhibited a 15% decrease in blood pressure compared to the placebo group."

      Past tense ("received", "exhibited") for specific observations and findings

6. **Discussion**:
    - **Interpretation of results**: Present tense when discussing the implications of the results.
    - **Comparison with previous research**: Present tense when discussing established knowledge; past tense when referring to specific studies or findings.
    - **Limitations**: Present or past tense, depending on whether the limitation is ongoing or was specific to the study.
    - **Conclusions or recommendations**: Present tense when extrapolating the findings to broader contexts or making suggestions for future research.

      Example: "Drug X reduces blood pressure effectively. Smith et al. (2010) found similar results with a related compound. However, our study did not account for diet variations, which may influence results."

Present tense ("reduces") for implications or general statements.

Past tense ("found") when referencing specific past studies.

Past tense ("did not account") for specific actions or limitations of the present study.

7. **Conclusion**:

- A mix of past tense when referencing the study's specific findings and present tense when discussing the broader implications or significance of those findings.

    Example: "Our research demonstrated that Drug X offers a promising avenue for hypertension treatment. Further research is required for long-term effects."

    Past tense ("demonstrated") for specific study findings.

    Present tense ("offers", "is required") for ongoing implications or recommendations

8. **Figures and Tables**:

- Legends and captions: Typically past tense, as they describe data collected or analyses performed. Legend

Example: "Figure 1: Blood pressure levels before and after Drug X administed."

Past tense ("administered") referring to data collection during the study.

In addition to these general guidelines, it's essential to maintain consistency within sections. The clarity of writing in a research paper is of utmost importance. Being mindful of tense usage will help ensure that the findings and discussions are presented as clearly and unambiguously as possible.

# CHAPTER 11

# Advice to Beginners for Writing a Research Paper

**TOPIC OUTLINE**

- How much data does a full research paper require?
- Logical and straightforward presentation
- Information relevance
- A rule of thumb
- Presentation

## How Much Data Does a Full Research Paper Require?

A research paper should be a complete story but not a truncated document. It should completely address the questions raised in the proposal. Generally, the higher the impact of the journal, the more results are required. Before submitting the work for publication, you should check the journal instructions about the word limits and figure and table allowance.

*Data quality:* You must check the outcome qualities, including sample size, statistical methods, significance levels, and effect size.

*Research design:* Is the research design appropriate to address the question? Are the questions descriptive, different, associative, or causal? A good research project should have novelty, be excellent quality, and be systematic.

Writing a research paper, especially for beginners, can be a daunting task. The content and quality of data are paramount. Here's an elaboration on your excellent pointers, and a few additional tips for beginners:

1. **Scope of the Study**: It's essential to understand that a research paper should not be too broad or too narrow. Having a defined scope allows you to keep your research focused and relevant.

   **Example**: If you're researching the effects of caffeine on cognitive function, you might narrow your scope to "the effects of caffeine on short-term memory in adults aged 18-25."

   **Explanation**: This refined scope prevents the study from becoming too broad (e.g., studying all cognitive functions in all age groups) and ensures that the research is manageable and specific.

2. **Quality Over Quantity**: It's far better to have fewer, high-quality, well-interpreted data than to have pages of inconclusive or irrelevant results. Thoroughly analyze and understand every piece of data you include.

   **Example**: Instead of presenting 100 vaguely related results to a hypothesis, present 20 directly relevant, thoroughly analyzed results.

   **Explanation**: An abundance of irrelevant data can cloud the primary objective of your research. Always ensure that every data point has a clear and direct relevance to your research questions.

3. **Research Design**: It's crucial to ensure that your research design aligns with your questions. The design will dictate the type of data you need and the methodology you use.

   **Example**: If you're asking whether one variable causes a change in another (e.g., does caffeine consumption cause an increase in short-term memory?), you'll need an experimental research design with control and experimental groups.

   **Explanation**: An experimental design can help establish causation, while other designs (like observational studies) can only suggest correlation.

4. **Replicability**: Other researchers should be able to replicate your study using the methods you've described. This means that you should provide enough detail about how you collected and analyzed your data.

   **Example**: If you used a specific brand and dosage of caffeine pills for your study, mention that exact brand and dosage.

   **Explanation**: Such specifics ensure that another researcher can replicate your study under the same conditions to verify the results.

5. **Literature Review**: Make sure to conduct an exhaustive literature review. Understand the existing research in your field to identify gaps, which your research aims to

fill. This will provide a foundation and context for your study.

**Example**: Previous studies might have found that caffeine improves attention and alertness. However, its effects on short-term memory might be less studied, creating a research gap.

**Explanation**: Knowing what has been studied helps you identify what hasn't, guiding your research's direction and significance.

6. **Clarity and Organization**: Your paper should be well-organized with clear headings, subheadings, and flow. The reader should be able to follow your line of thought without getting lost.

7. **Discussion and Conclusion**: Ensure you don't just present data. Analyze it. Discuss its implications, how it fits in with or contradicts existing research, and what new questions it might raise.

   **Example**: If your data shows that caffeine significantly improves short-term memory, compare this with previous studies. Maybe older studies had contrasting results, or perhaps your results add more nuance to the current understanding.

   **Explanation**: This section contextualizes your findings within the broader academic conversation, offering insights and interpretations beyond the raw data.

8. **Feedback**: Before submitting, get feedback from peers, mentors, or experts in your field. They can offer insights you might have missed and point out any potential weaknesses in your paper.
9. **Ethical Considerations**: If your research involves humans, animals, or sensitive data, ensure you've followed all ethical guidelines and obtained necessary permissions or consents.
10. **Proofreading and Editing**: This cannot be stressed enough. A well-written paper is more likely to be accepted. Ensure there are no grammatical errors, and your writing is clear and concise. Use tools or professional services if necessary.

Writing a research paper is a meticulous process that requires a balance of quality data, clear writing, and a thorough understanding of your field. The key is to remain patient, diligent, and passionate about your research topic.

## Logical and Straightforward Presentation

Writing is an art, but most importantly, it needs to be accurate and concise. The story flow must be logical, with ideas having a critical starting point, the main content, an explanation, and a conclusion. You need to choose where to start carefully, follow step-by-step in a logical order, and avoid having ideas jumping around.

Usually, it is a good idea to start a paragraph with an acceptable concept, a hypothesis, or a model that helps a reader quickly grab and accept the idea. After you have presented the idea, the writing should not stop and leave the reader to work it out. Instead, you should explain and provide critical information, for example, considering relevant structure or anatomy, physiology, injury, and intervention. Remember that you want the reader to understand the idea and follow the presentation without an extra reading of the literature or scientific background.

Let's delve into the specifics of presenting information logically and straightforwardly.

1. **Logical Sequence**:
    - **Example**: When discussing the development of a new drug, one might start with the identification of a medical problem, followed by target identification, drug design, preclinical testing, and then stages of clinical trials.
    - **Explanation**: This sequence reflects the actual process of drug development, making it easier for readers to follow.

2. **Presenting Data Clearly**:
    - **Example**: If you're discussing the effects of a drug on cell growth, a well-labeled graph showing cell numbers over time for treated vs. untreated groups will be more effective than just a textual description.
    - **Explanation**: Visual representations can often clarify complex datasets, allowing the reader to see trends and patterns more clearly.

3. **Avoid Overcomplication**:
    - **Example**: While explaining a molecular pathway, focus on the major players and reactions instead of delving into every possible minor interaction.
    - **Explanation**: Providing too much detail can confuse readers, making them lose sight of the primary focus.

4. **Connect the Dots for the Reader**:
    - **Example**: After presenting the data, explicitly state what it means. For instance, "The increased expression of Protein Y in treated cells indicates that Drug X activates its pathway."
    - **Explanation**: While the data may seem self-explanatory, directly stating the implications ensures clarity.

5. **Use Analogies or Metaphors**:
    - **Example**: If explaining a complex mechanism, such as DNA replication, you might compare it to the process of unzipping and copying a set of instructions.
    - **Explanation**: Analogies can bridge the gap between complex scientific concepts and more familiar ideas.

6. **Avoid Jargon or Clearly Define It**:

- **Example**: If discussing a "polygenic risk score," provide a brief definition or simplify the term if possible.
- **Explanation**: Jargon can alienate readers who aren't specialists in that particular subfield.

7. **Progress from Basic to Advanced Ideas**:
    - **Example**: Before delving into the nuances of a specific signaling pathway, give an overview of the cell types and broader physiological context involved.
    - **Explanation**: By building on foundational knowledge, the reader is better prepared to understand advanced concepts.

8. **Use Headers and Subheaders**:
    - **Example**: In a paper about the cardiovascular effects of a drug, use clear headings like "Effect on Blood Pressure," "Impact on Heart Rate," and "Vascular Responses."
    - **Explanation**: Headings provide structure, helping readers navigate the content and focus on areas of interest.

9. **Summarize and Conclude**:

- **Example**: After presenting the various effects of a drug, provide a summary section detailing the drug's overall efficacy and potential clinical implications.
- **Explanation**: This encapsulates the primary messages, reinforcing them for the reader.

By ensuring that the presentation of information is both logical and straightforward, researchers and writers can effectively communicate complex topics, enhancing understanding and fostering collaboration in the scientific community.

## Information Relevance

Information relevance in the context of biomedical research papers pertains to the degree to which the information presented in a paper is pertinent, meaningful, and valuable to the reader's specific needs, objectives, or interests. Given the vast and expanding volume of biomedical literature, determining the relevance of a particular piece of information or a full paper becomes crucial for researchers, clinicians, students, policymakers, and other stakeholders in the biomedical field.

Here are several key aspects:

1. **Research Question and Objectives**: The relevance of information is often gauged by how well it aligns with the reader's research question or objectives. For

example, a clinical trial studying the effects of a new drug on hypertension might not be relevant to a researcher interested in the molecular mechanisms of Alzheimer's disease.

2. **Recency**: In rapidly evolving fields, the most recent information might be seen as more relevant than older findings. For instance, a therapeutic strategy proposed a decade ago might be less pertinent today due to advances in technology or new discoveries.

3. **Methodological Rigor**: The validity and reliability of the research methodology can affect its relevance. If a study is poorly designed or has significant flaws, its findings might not be considered relevant, regardless of the topic.

4. **Population and Setting**: A study's relevance can be influenced by the population under investigation and the setting. For example, results from animal models might not be directly relevant to human diseases, or findings in one ethnic group might not apply universally.

5. **Impact Factor and Journal Reputation**: While not a perfect metric, the impact factor and reputation of the journal in which the paper is published can give an indication of the paper's significance and relevance in the field.

6. **Citations**: A paper that is frequently cited by other researchers in the field can be an indicator of its relevance and impact.

7. **Abstract and Keywords**: The abstract and keywords of a research paper provide a snapshot of its content. Researchers often scan these sections first to gauge the paper's relevance to their work.

## Guidelines for Biomedical Research Paper Writing:

- Text should clearly convey intricate concepts and detail the findings of the study.
- Figures should be employed to underscore major findings, particularly those indicating noteworthy shifts or changes.
- Tables are recommended for summarizing and presenting extensive datasets in a comprehensible manner.

## Considering Rapid Publication? Here's What to Know:

It's always more advantageous to publish a thorough and complete study rather than rushing to release an "incomplete work." However, there may be circumstances when a researcher contemplates a swift publication. In such cases, presenting at a conference is a preferable route. This approach ensures that you retain the potential to publish the data comprehensively as a full paper later on.

Remember, it's unethical to "double-dip" in publications. Any data submitted for publication should be original and not previously published elsewhere.

## Effective Time Allocation for Crafting a Research Paper:

Drafting a research paper necessitates judicious time management. Here's a suggested breakdown for allocating your time:

- **Research Foundation (40%)**: This includes identifying the research objective, grasping the core topic, and conducting a literature review.
- **Study Design (10%)**: Dedicate time to brainstorm the experimental methodology and design your research study.
- **Experiment Execution (40%)**: The actual conducting of experiments or data gathering should form a significant chunk of your time.
- **Paper Composition (10%)**: Allocate the remaining time to the writing process, ensuring clarity and cohesion in your report.

While this framework provides a general guideline, it's important to note that individual preferences and workflows can cause variations in time allocation.

PART FIVE

# Examples

**TOPIC OUTLINE**

- Abstract examples
- Introduction examples
- Method examples
- Table examples
- Figure examples

# Abstract Examples

## A Case-Control Association Study

*Features:* A structured abstract uses background, methods, results, and conclusions to summarize the study. A case-control study examines the differences between treatments and the association between variables.

*Writing skills:* The sequence is to present (1) the knowns and unknowns, (2) subjects and measures, (3) results, and (4) conclusions and significance.

***Examples:***

*Background:* Evidence indicates that the serum concentration of uric acid relates to the pathophysiology and therapeutics of bipolar disorder (BPD). This study aimed to examine serum UA concentration changes and clinical significance in first-episode manic patients suffering from BPD.

*#Comments: Indicating what is known and unknown.*

Methods: Seventy-six drug-naive patients with first-episode bipolar mania and seventy-six age- and gender-matched healthy subjects were recruited. Young Mania Rating Scale and Hamilton Depression Rating Scale were used to assess clinical symptoms. We tested serum UA concentrations by immunosorbent assay at baseline and at the end of 8-week treatment in BPD patients and controls.

*#Comments: The experimental design introduces subjects and measures.*

Results: After 8-week drug treatment, this study revealed that the serum UA concentrations in remitted patients were significantly lower than in non-remitted patients; however, those remitted patients still had higher serum UA than healthy controls. We discovered that the baseline UA concentration was higher in non-remitted than remitted patients after eight weeks of treatment. Finally, a positive association was found between serum UA and symptom relief in the first episode of manic disorder patients.

*#Comments: Results include the low, high, and association analysis.*

Conclusion: Patients with first-episode BPD had high serum UA levels, which respond to treatment mainly in remitted patients. Our results suggest that serum UA concentrations might present a trait marker in bipolar patients.

*#Comments: Conclusion and significance are described.*

*Extracted and modified from a paper:* "Patients with Drug-Naïve Bipolar Disorder in Remission After Eight Weeks of Treatment Had Decreased Serum Uric Acid Concentrations" (Chen et al., 2019) with modifications.

## A Cell- and Animal-Based Intervention

*Features:* The abstract summarizes the studies, why to investigate, how to do it, and the findings and why they are important.

*Writing skills:* The presentation starts with known/unknown, intervention/measurement, increased/induced/reduced, and conclusion.

### *Example:*

Background: The approved small-molecule drug ibrutinib *effectively targeted* patients with chronic lymphocytic leukemia. Ibrutinib *inhibits* Bruton's tyrosine kinase. However, ibrutinib has not comprehensively examined the regulation of neuroinflammatory responses in the brain.

*#Comments: Describes what we know and do not know.*

Methods: Microglial cells *were* treated with ibrutinib or vehicle, followed by lipopolysaccharide (LPS) or vehicle. RT-PCR, immunocytochemistry, and subcellular fractionation were performed to examine the effects of ibrutinib on neuroinflammatory responses. Wild-type mice were injected with ibrutinib or vehicle, followed by LPS or vehicle, and microglial and astrocyte activations were assessed using immunohistochemistry.

*#Comments: Describes research design (intervention) and measurement. The method section used past simple passive tense.*

Results: Ibrutinib significantly reduced LPS-induced increases in proinflammatory cytokine levels in BV2 microglial and primary microglial cells but not in primary astrocytes. Ibrutinib significantly decreased LPS-induced increases in p-AKT and p-STAT3 levels, suggesting that ibrutinib attenuates LPS-induced neuroinflammatory responses by inhibiting AKT/STAT3 signalling pathways. Moreover, ibrutinib-injected wild-type mice exhibited significantly *reduced* microglial activation.

*#Comments: The results describe what was reduced or decreased. A decrease followed by suggestions points out possible mechanisms.*

Conclusions: Our data *provides* insights into the mechanisms of a potential therapeutic strategy for neuroinflammation-related diseases.

*#Comments: The conclusion provides the mechanism. The significance describes therapeutic strategy.*

*Extracted and modified from a paper:* "Ibrutinib Suppresses LPS-Induced Neuroinflammatory Responses in BV2 Microglial Cells and Wild-Type Mice" (Nam et al., 2018).

## Working Flow Sequence

*Features:* A one-paragraph unstructured abstract presents the motivation of the study, establishes an experimental model followed by interventions, identifies causes responsible for the problem, and moves on to another animal model for further confirmation.

*Writing skills:* The contents include (1) what is known and the problem, (2) models used, (3) results of methods, and (4) conclusions and significance.

### *Example:*

Antipsychotic drugs ***are*** **used** to treat psychiatric disorders ***but*** are associated with significant weight gain and metabolic disease.

*#Comments: States the application and problem.*

Increased food intake **appears** to be a driving force by which antipsychotics induce weight gain, **but** the mechanisms *are* poorly understood.

*#Comments: Points out the problem and unknown mechanism.*

Here we report that the administration of antipsychotics to *C. elegans* **induces** hyperphagia by a mechanism that **is** genetically distinct from basal food intake.

*#Comments: Explains the meaning of the results.*

We exploit this finding to screen for adjuvant drugs that *suppress* antipsychotics-induced hyperphagia in *C. elegans* and mice.

*#Comments: Performs a follow-up study.*

In mice, AP-induced hyperphagia is associated with a hypothalamic gene expression that is abolished by adjuvant drug treatment. Genetic analysis using *C. elegans identifies* two transcription factors required for AP-induced hyperphagia.

*#Comments: Proves the finding using another mode.*

Our study *reveals* that AP-induced hyperphagia **can** be selectively suppressed without affecting basal food intake, allowing for novel drug discovery **strategies** *to* combat AP-induced metabolic side effects.

*#Comments: Provides conclusion remark and significance*

*Extracted and modified from a paper:* "A Phenotypic *Caenorhabditis Elegans* Screen Identifies a Selective Suppressor of Antipsychotic-Induced Hyperphagia" (Perez-Gomez et al., 2018).

## One Focus

*Features:* The abstract has only one focus, e.g., Urolithin A, UA. The abstract presents the molecular mechanism and functions using various models with this focus.

*Writing skills:* The contents include (1) what is known and the problem, (2) models used, (3) results of methods, and (4) conclusions and significance.

### *Example:*

The biological effects of urolithins **remain** poorly characterized, despite widespread human **exposure** via the dietary consumption of their metabolic precursors found in pomegranate fruit, nuts, and berries.

*#Comments: States this is a molecule with poor characterizations, although there are widespread applications.*

We found urolithin A as a natural compound that induces mitophagy in vitro and in vivo. In *C. elegans*, UA prevented the accumulation of dysfunctional mitochondria with age and extended lifespan. Furthermore, urolithin A **prolonged** activity during aging in *C. elegans*, including mobility and pharyngeal pumping, while maintaining mitochondrial respiratory capacity.

*#Comments: Reports that the testing molecule has several functions.*

These effects translated to rodents, where urolithin A **improved** exercise capacity in two different mouse models of age-related decline of muscle function in rats.

*#Comments: Confirms the benefits in other models.*

Our findings **highlight** the health benefits of urolithin A and its potential **application** in strategies to improve mitochondrial and muscle function.

*#Comments: Provides conclusion and significance.*

*Extracted and modified from a paper:* "Urolithin A Induces Mitophagy and Prolongs Lifespan in C. Elegans and Increases Muscle Function in Rodents" (Ryu et al., 2016).

## Focuses on a Story

*Features:* This abstract uses a qualitative rather than quantitative approach to describe a story about a problem via several steps to its results. Choosing the suitable biomarkers to address the questions is a strength of this paper, e.g., hypothalamic cytokines, gliosis, and MRI measures.

*Writing skills:* Raise a problem, present results, and then conclude.

***Example:***

Rodent models of obesity induced by consuming a high-fat diet (HFD) **are** characterized by inflammation in both peripheral tissues and hypothalamic areas critical for energy homeostasis.

*#Comments: Points out the problem.*

Here, we **report** that unlike inflammation in peripheral tissues, which develops due to obesity, hypothalamic inflammatory signaling was evident in both rats and mice within 1 to 3 days of HFD onset, prior to substantial weight gain.

*#Comments: Reports new findings with a comparison.*

Furthermore, both reactive gliosis and markers suggestive of neuron injury were evident in the hypothalamic arcuate nucleus of rats and mice within the first week of HFD feeding.

*#Comments: Describe the findings in chronological order.*

Although these responses temporarily subsided, suggesting that neuroprotective mechanisms may initially limit the damage, with continued HFD feeding, inflammation and gliosis returned permanently to the mediobasal hypothalamus.

*#Comments: Describes the time effect and shows a defensive*

*response.*

Consistent with these data in rodents, we found evidence of increased gliosis in the mediobasal hypothalamus of obese humans, as assessed by MRI.

*#Comments: Adds human data.*

These findings collectively suggest that obesity is associated with neuronal injury in a brain area crucial for body weight control in both human and rodent models.

*#Comments: Provides conclusion remark.*

*Extracted and modified from a paper:* "Obesity Is Associated with Hypothalamic Injury in Rodents and Humans" (Thaler et al., 2012).

## A Single Receptor with Several Characterizations

*Features:* An abstract emphasizes the story or qualitative data presentation. There is only one focus, GPR120, with several studies to characterize it.

*Writing skills:* The presentation starts with known versus unknown, then provides the results and conclusion.

### ***Example:***

Omega-3 fatty acids (n-3 FAs), DHA, and EPA **exert** anti-inflammatory effects, but the mechanisms **are** poorly understood.

*#Comments: Points out what we know and don't know.*

Here we show that GPR120 functions as an n-3 FA receptor. Stimulation of GPR120 with n-3 FAs or a chemical agonist causes broad anti-inflammatory effects in monocytic cells and primary intraperitoneal macrophages. All of these effects are abrogated by GPR120 knockdown.

*#Comments: Results are qualitative instead of quantitative from receptor characterization, stimulation, and knockout studies. The author uses the receptor as the center and describes several aspects.*

Since chronic macrophage-mediated tissue inflammation **is** a key mechanism for insulin resistance in obesity, we *fed* obese WT and GPR120 knockout mice a high-fat diet with or without n-3 FA supplementation. The n-3 FA treatment *inhibited* inflammation and *enhanced* systemic insulin sensitivity in normal mice but was without effect in GPR120 knockout mice.

*#Comments: Uses in vivo model to prove the concept.*

In conclusion, GPR120 is a functional ω-3 FA receptor/sensor and mediates potent insulin-sensitizing and antidiabetic effects in vivo by repressing macrophage-induced tissue inflammation.

*#Comments: Provides conclusion remarks.*

*Extracted and modified from a paper:* "GPR120 Is an Omega-3 Fatty Acid Receptor Mediating Potent Anti-Inflammatory and Insulin-Sensitizing Effects" (Oh et al., 2010).

# Introduction Examples

## An Association Study

*Features:* This introduction starts with the research topic, gap, broad relevance, and research questions, followed by findings.

*Writing skills:* The presentation sequence is the research topic, gap/justification, findings, and conclusion.

***Example:***

Obesity has emerged as a major health problem in industrialized nations. Despite substantial progress in understanding the neurobiology of energy homeostasis, little is known regarding how brain systems designed to promote weight stability are altered in common forms of obesity.

*#Comments: Introduces the research topic and gap.*

Growing evidence implicates immune cell-mediated tissue inflammation as an important mechanism linking obesity to insulin resistance in metabolically active organs, such as the liver, skeletal muscle, and adipose tissue.

*#Comments: States broad relevance.*

In rodent diet-induced obesity, increased inflammatory signalling in the hypothalamus contributes to leptin resistance and weight gain, but the cellular interactions underlying this inflammatory response remain uncharacterized. This study aims to identify the neuroanatomical correlates of obesity-associated hypothalamic inflammation and to determine whether similar responses occur in humans.

*#Comments: States the research question and aim.*

We report that unlike inflammation in peripheral tissues, a process that develops over months of high-fat diet (HFD) feeding in rodents, markers of hypothalamic inflammation are elevated within 24 hours of HFD exposure. Within the first week, markers of neuron injury become evident in the arcuate nucleus in association with reactive gliosis involving the recruitment of both microglia and astrocytes. Although initially transient, suggesting an effective neuroprotective response, inflammation and gliosis return and become established with continued HFD exposure. Using MRI, we also report evidence of increased gliosis in the hypothalamus of obese humans. These findings collectively suggest that, in both humans and rodents, obesity is associated with injury to a brain area for energy homeostasis.

*#Comments: Reports the results.*

*Extracted and modified from a paper:* "Obesity Is Associated with Hypothalamic Injury in Rodents and Humans" (Thaler et al., 2012).

# Method Examples

## A Retrospective Case-Control Study

*Features:* The method requires detailed records of the cases and control subjects to evaluate external validity by readers.

*Writing skill:* The research design describes the details of the subjects involved and treated. The detailed elements are essential, as this type of clinical study could have many variations.

***Example:***

This project recruited 76 patients with bipolar disorders from 2015 to 2017 from Beijing Hospital. The inclusion criteria were subjects between 18 and 45 years old with a diagnosis of a manic or hypomanic episode by qualified psychiatrists. The study did not include subjects with a history of affective disorder, schizophrenia, and neurological illness. In addition, researchers recruited comparable healthy controls from the local community. All subjects had informed consent approved by the institutional ethics committee.

*#Comments: Describes the patients, time, location, criteria, controls, and consent.*

All patients received the combination quetiapine (606.58 ± 150.85 mg daily) plus sodium valproate (1,077.97 ± 338.77 mg daily) treatment for eight weeks.

*#Comments: Describe the treatment drugs and duration.*

*Extracted and modified from a paper:* "Patients with Drug-Naïve Bipolar Disorder in Remission After Eight Weeks of Treatment Had Decreased Serum Uric Acid Concentrations" (Chen et al., 2019).

## Clinical Assessment

*Features:* The method provides how, when, and by whom the clinical assessment was performed and uses correlation coefficient analysis to ensure rating reliability between researchers.

*Writing skill: Keeping the key elements relevant to the study.*

***Example:***

Psychopathological symptoms of patients were assessed on the day of blood sampling by four psychiatrists who were blind to the clinical status and treatment conditions. Young Mania Rating Scale (YMRS) was used to measure the severity of manic symptoms before and after treatment.

*#Comments: Describes when, who, and how.*

To ensure consistency and reliability of ratings, before undertaking the study, four psychiatrists who worked over five years in clinical practice simultaneously received a training session on how to use YMRS, ensuring a correlation coefficient maintained greater than 0.8 by repeated assessments across the study.

*#Comments: Uses a correlation coefficient > 0.8 between psychiatrists to ensure rating reliability.*

*Extracted and modified from a paper:* "Patients with Drug-Naïve Bipolar Disorder in Remission After Eight Weeks of Treatment Had Decreased Serum Uric Acid Concentrations" (Chen et al., 2019).

## Laboratory Tests

*Features:* The method describes what and how the parameters were measured, including the samples, procedures, criteria, and possible confounding factors.

*Writing skill:* Provides detailed techniques, measurements, and criteria appropriate to support research aims.

### *Example:*

The blood samples from all subjects were taken between 6, and 7 am after overnight fasting as baseline eight weeks after treatments.

*#Comments: Describes the sample collection.*

Serum uric acid concentrations were assessed using a sandwich enzyme-linked immunosorbent assay, a commercially available kit (DRG kit, Germany).

*#Comments: Describes the measurement kit used.*

The parameters potentially affecting serum uric acid concentrations such as metabolic parameters (triglycerides, high-density lipoprotein cholesterol, and fasting blood glucose) and kidney function (creatinine, urea) were also measured.

*#Comments: Identifies confounders relevant to the study.*

The height, body weight, and blood pressure of all subjects were measured. Body mass index was calculated. Hyperuricemia was defined as serum level of uric acid >420 μmol/l (7.0 mg/dl) for men and >360 μmol/l (6.0 mg/dl) for women (17). Current smoking refers to smoking at least one cigarette per day over the last one month before enrollment.

*#Comments: Provides participants' demographic data, diagnosis*

*criteria, and the possible confounder, smoking.*

*Extracted and modified from a paper:* "Patients with Drug-Naïve Bipolar Disorder in Remission After Eight Weeks of Treatment Had Decreased Serum Uric Acid Concentrations" (Chen et al., 2019).

## Statistical Analysis for a Clinical Study

*Features:* The method explains what statistical tests were used and why they were chosen.

*Writing skills:* Provides the difference, association, normality, and covariant.

***Example:***

The differences in demographic data between patients and controls were analyzed by $\chi2$ test or independent-samples t-test, wherever appropriate. The paired *t*-test *was* used to compare serum uric acid concentrations between the baseline and posttreatment in the patient group. Independent-samples *t*-test was applied to single-time-point data. When significant differences were detected, covariant analysis controlling for BMI, age, and sex and Bonferroni post hoc analyses for multiple comparisons were applied.

*#Comments: Describes statistical tests for the differences with justifications.*

Pearson correlation coefficient was used to evaluate the relationship between serum uric acid levels and YMRS scores when data *were* in a normal distribution.

*#Comments: Uses the Pearson test for analyzing association.*

Results are expressed as mean ± SD. All statistical tests were two-tailed, and $p < 0.05$ was considered statistically significant. Statistical analyses were performed using SPSS (version 17.0).

*Extracted and modified from a paper:* "Patients with Drug-Naïve Bipolar Disorder in Remission After Eight Weeks of Treatment

Had Decreased Serum Uric Acid Concentrations" (Chen et al., 2019).

## Statistical Analysis for a Laboratory Study

*Features:* The method should provide why you have used those statistical tests.

*Writing skill:* When describing the statistical test, you may combine it with the purpose.

### *Example:*

Survival analyses were performed using the Kaplan Meier method, and the significance of differences between survival curves was calculated using the log-rank test. Shapiro-Wilk normality test was used to assess the normal distribution of the samples when appropriate ($n > 8$).

*#Comments: Uses Kaplan Meier test for survival analysis and Shapiro-Wilk test for data normality.*

Differences between the two groups were assessed using two-tailed *t*-tests. Differences between more than two groups were assessed by using one-way ANOVA. Two-way ANOVA tests were performed to compare the interaction between the two factors. Analysis of variance, assessed by Bonferroni's multiple-comparison test, was used when comparing more than two groups.

*#Comments: Tests the differences.*

R (R software version 2.9.0) was used for calculating mean lifespan and s.e.m., and GraphPad Prism 5 (GraphPad Software) was used for all other statistical analyses. All *p*-values <0.05 were considered to be significant. $*p \leq 0.05$; $**p \leq 0.01$; $***P \leq 0.001$ instead stated otherwise.

All animal experiments were performed once. Animals that showed signs of severity predefined by the animal authorization were euthanized. These animals and those who died spontaneously during the experiments were excluded from the calculations. These criteria were established before starting the experiments.

In Figure 6, two outliers (control) not following the normal distribution of the samples were removed based on a Shapiro–Wilk normality test.

For lifespan experiments in *C. elegans*, the sample size was determined as previously. For all other experiments, the sample size was estimated based on the known variability of the assay. All experiments were done non-blinded.

*Extracted and modified from a paper:* "Urolithin A Induces Mitophagy and Prolongs Lifespan in *C. elegans*, and Increases Muscle Function In Rodents" (Ryu et al., 2016).

# Discussion Examples

## The First Paragraph

*Features:* You should describe the main point, story, and conclusion.

*Writing skill:* The first paragraph of the discussion can start with the *main point* by saying what is known and unknown, then provide the *specific findings using* the *time sequence* and presenting them as a logical story, and finally land on a conclusion.

***Example:***

Although hypothalamic inflammation is well documented in rodent models of diet-induced obesity, neither its underlying mechanisms nor its relevance to human obesity is understood. Here, we report that hypothalamic inflammation induced by a high-fat diet (HFD) is a manifestation of neuron injury that in turn triggers reactive gliosis involving both microglial and astroglial cell populations.

*#Comments: Raises the question and provides the answer.*

Moreover, these responses appear selectively in the hypothalamic arcuate nucleus and rapidly follow the initiation of an HFD. The transient nature of this hypothalamic response suggests that neuroprotective responses are mounted that limit or reverse the injury during its initial phases, but with sustained exposure to the HFD, ARC gliosis and injury responses are re-established.

*#Comments: Describes the study with details and specificity.*

Combined with MRI-based evidence for gliosis in the MBH of obese humans, our findings suggest that, in both humans and rodent DIO models, obesity is associated with neuron injury in a brain area crucial for body weight control.

*#Comments: Provides the conclusion.*

*Extracted and modified from a paper:* "Obesity Is Associated with Hypothalamic Injury in Rodents and Humans" (Thaler et al., 2012).

## Taking Our Knowledge a Step Further

*Features:* By laying out what we know, the discussion delivers the findings, the new concept that advanced our knowledge.

*Writing skill:* The author proves the advancement of knowledge using the existing knowledge as a basis. Then, the author provides new findings, cites supporting evidence from the literature, and summarizes the meaning of the discovery.

### *Example:*

Several mechanisms have been forwarded to explain obesity-induced inflammation in both peripheral tissues and the hypothalamus (ref). While the contribution made by these mechanisms remains uncertain, the much earlier onset of inflammation in the hypothalamus relative to that in peripheral tissues raises the possibility that different processes are involved.

*#Comments: Describes what is known and what has been discovered.*

Moreover, the nature of the hypothalamic inflammation occurring during the first days of HFD feeding may differ fundamentally from that involved with chronic HFD exposure. The conclusion that the rapid onset of MBH inflammation is a manifestation of neuron injury and associated neuroprotective responses is consistent with previous evidence of apoptosis and glial ensheathment of ARC neurons in animals rendered obese by chronic HFD feeding (ref). Moreover, these responses were detected specifically in ARC POMC cells, which is consistent with our finding of an approximately 25% reduction in the number of hypothalamic POMC neurons in mice chronically fed a HFD (ref).

*#Comments: Describes new findings and supporting reference (ref).*

In this context, it is noteworthy that POMC cells play an essential role in protecting against obesity and that loss of these cells is sufficient in and of itself to cause excess weight gain in mice.

*#Comments: Summarizes the meaning of the outcomes.*

*Extracted and modified from a paper:* "Obesity Is Associated with Hypothalamic Injury in Rodents and Humans" (Thaler et al., 2012).

## Develop a New Concept

*Features:* The discussion shows how to develop a new concept by providing evidence of the pathology development over time.

*Writing skill:* Current knowledge plus new findings with a supporting reference lead to a new concept.

***Example:***

In experimental models of brain injury, astrocytes play a key neuroprotective role, limiting the extent of both inflammation and neuron loss (refs).

*#Comments: Describes current knowledge.*

The reactive gliosis we observed in the hypothalamus of rats and mice may therefore be neuroprotective, limiting local injury induced by high-fat diet feeding. Consistent with this hypothesis is our finding that the return of proinflammatory markers in the hypothalamus to basal level on day 7 of a high-fat diet coincides with the appearance of reactive gliosis in the same area. Like markers of inflammation, however, this gliosis is initially transient, but both responses are re-established as obesity develops with a continued high-fat diet.

*#Comments: Explains the chronological events.*

These observations suggest that with sustained exposure, the capacity of supportive glial cells to control the damage associated with HFD feeding is exceeded and that neuron *injury and loss* can no longer be prevented.

*#Comments: Describes a new concept.*

*Extracted and modified from a paper:* "Obesity Is Associated with Hypothalamic Injury in Rodents and Humans" (Thaler et al., 2012).

## Results Differ from the Literature

*Features:* The discussion should provide a summary paragraph if there are discrepancies between the new findings and previous data. Clinical research can produce very different data, even having a similar research design. When discussing, you may weigh the quality and significance of each article, cite the relevant literature, and then do a summary and give your opinion.

*Writing skill:* Cite all relevant papers available and give your opinion.

***Example:***

The prevalence of metabolic syndrome in bipolar patients varies significantly from 8.5 to 67% from study to study reported in the literature.

*#Comments: Points out the issue: a large variation.*

A high prevalence (67%) was reported in an Australian study and 53% prevalence in an Indian study in bipolar patients suffering from metabolic syndrome. On the other hand, a low prevalence of metabolic syndrome in bipolar patients was reported in French (18.5%) and Spanish (22.4%) studies (refs). In addition, two other Indian studies report that the prevalence of metabolic syndrome in bipolar patients is about 40%, similar to the 42% found in this study. On the other hand, the prevalence of metabolic syndrome in control subjects was 21.9% in the present study, which was similar to previous Chinese studies on the normal population (24.5%).

*#Comments: Lists the details.*

The possible explanation for such significant discrepancies may be due to the different ethnicities, regions, dietary habits, and genetic backgrounds of the patients investigated.

*#Comments: Gives a possible explanation.*

*Extracted and modified from a paper:* "Association between Hyperuricemia and Metabolic Syndrome in Patients Who Have Bipolar Disorder" (An et al., 2015).

## Similar Results to the Literature

*Features:* The discussion should point out the research outcome similarities between your study and others'. You can start with your findings, cite other studies, make comparisons for similarities and differences, and then draw a conclusion.

*Writing skill:* The content provides the results, literature data, justification, and significance.

***Example:***

Our results confirmed that serum uric acid concentrations in bipolar patients were significantly higher than in healthy controls (ref).

*#Comments: Confirms the results.*

Animal study shows that uric acid induces endothelial dysfunction and overproduction of reactive oxygen species, which has been considered a major factor of insulin resistance. In humans, hyperuricemia is also associated with insulin resistance and metabolic syndrome.

*#Comments: Points out the disease's relevance.*

Therefore, elevated uric acid worse insulin sensitivity and metabolic syndrome and *vice versa*. Both hyperuricemia and metabolic syndrome increase the risk of cardiovascular disease and dementia in older adults. However, ageing is not necessarily associated with increased blood uric acid. This study showed that bipolar patients with hyperuricemia and over 50 years of age have a very high prevalence of metabolic disorders and their components. Therefore, particular caution should be taken to prevent cardiovascular diseases when there is hyperuricemia in elderly bipolar patients.

| |
|---|
| *#Comments: Raises specific concerns.* |

*Extracted and modified from a paper:* "Association between Hyperuricemia and Metabolic Syndrome in Patients Who Have Bipolar Disorder" (Chen et al., 2018).

## Limitations

*Features:* The discussion always has a paragraph or several sentences at the end of the article to describe limitations, especially if it is clinical research. Many variations in clinical research can contribute to the outcomes, e.g., sample size, gender, geography, ethnicity, study duration, participant recruitment time, and instrument accuracy.

*Writing skill:* Identifies the limitations relevant to the study aim, including unpredictable conditions and confounding factors.

***Example:***

This study has some limitations.

First, only the inpatients with bipolar disorder were included, who tend to suffer more severely, have more comorbidities, and have higher rates of pharmacological treatment than outpatients. Therefore, our data do not necessarily reflect the prevalence of metabolic syndrome in outpatients with bipolar disorder.

*#Comments: States that the study does not represent all patients.*

Second, antidepressant (e.g., mirtazapine) uses were not obtained in this study, which could cause weight gain and metabolic disorders (ref).

*#Comments: States the drug treatment limitations.*

Finally, other possible confounding factors were not ruled out, which could play a role in contributing to the development of metabolic syndrome, including types and duration of antipsychotic drugs used, diet, physical activity, socioeconomic status, and alcohol use.

| |
|---|
| *#Comments: Points out other confounders.* |

*Extracted and modified from a paper:* "Association between Hyperuricemia and Metabolic Syndrome in Patients Who Have Bipolar Disorder" (Chen et al., 2018).

# References

An, H., et al., 2018. "Serum NCAM Levels and Cognitive Deficits in First Episode Schizophrenia Patients versus Health Controls." *Schizophr Res.* 192, 457-458.

An, H.M., et al., 2015. "Altered IL-2, IL-6 and IL-8 Serum Levels in Schizophrenia Patients with Tardive Dyskinesia." *Schizophr Res.* 162, 261-8.

Barroga, E., Matanguihan, G.J., 2021. "Creating Logical Flow When Writing Scientific Articles." *J Korean Med Sci.* 36, e275.

Camer, D., Huang, X.F., 2014a. "Comment On: Oleanolic Acid Co-Administration Alleviates Ethanol-Induced Hepatic Injury via Nrf-2 and Ethanol-Metabolizing Modulation (Sic) in Rats." *Chem Biol Interact.* 223C, 116.

Camer, D., Huang, X.F., 2014b. "The Endothelin Pathway: A Protective or Detrimental Target of Bardoxolone Methyl on Cardiac Function in Patients with Advanced Chronic Kidney Disease?" *Am J Nephrol.* 40, 288-90.

Carpenter, W.T., Jr., Davis, J.M., 2012. "Another View of the History of Antipsychotic Drug Discovery and Development." *Mol Psychiatry.* 17, 1168-73.

Chen, J., et al., 2018. "Association between Hyperuricemia and Metabolic Syndrome in Patients Suffering from Bipolar Disorder." *BMC Psychiatry.* 18, 390.

Chen, J.X., et al., 2019. "Patients with Drug-Naive Bipolar Disorder in Remission after 8 Weeks of Treatment Had

Decreased Serum Uric Acid Concentrations." *Front Psychiatry*. 10, 767.

Chu, Y., et al., 2020. "Obesity Is Associated with Increased Severity of Disease in COVID-19 Pneumonia: A Systematic Review and Meta-Analysis." *Eur J Med Res*. 25, 64.

de Silva, V.A., et al., 2016. "Metformin in Prevention and Treatment of Antipsychotic Induced Weight Gain: A Systematic Review And Meta-Analysis." *BMC Psychiatry*. 16, 341.

Fonseka, T.M., Muller, D.J., Kennedy, S.H., 2016. "Inflammatory Cytokines and Antipsychotic-Induced Weight Gain: Review and Clinical Implications." *Mol Neuropsychiatry*. 2, 1-14.

Guan, J.S., et al., 2009. "HDAC2 Negatively Regulates Memory Formation and Synaptic Plasticity." *Nature*. 459, 55-60.

Huang, X.F., Chen, J.Z., 2009. "Obesity, the PI3K/AKT Signal Pathway and Colon Cancer." *Obes Rev*. 10, 610-6.

Huang, X.F., Song, X., 2019. "Effects of Antipsychotic Drugs on Neurites Relevant to Schizophrenia Treatment." *Med Res Rev*. 39, 386-403.

Kaur, J., 2014. "A Comprehensive Review on Metabolic Syndrome." *Cardiol Res Pract*. 2014, 943162.

Leucht, C., et al., 2011. "Oral Versus Depot Antipsychotic Drugs for Schizophrenia—A Critical Systematic Review and Meta-Analysis of Randomised Long-Term Trials." *Schizophr Res*. 127, 83-92.

Nam, H.Y., et al., 2018. "Ibrutinib Suppresses LPS-Induced Neuroinflammatory Responses in BV2 Microglial Cells and Wild-Type Mice." *J Neuroinflammation*. 15, 271.

Oh, D.Y., et al., 2010. GPR120 Is an Omega-3 Fatty Acid Receptor Mediating Potent Anti-Inflammatory and Insulin-Sensitizing Effects." *Cell.* 142, 687-98.

Park, J., et al., 2014. "Obesity and Cancer—Mechanisms Underlying Tumour Progression and Recurrence." *Nat Rev Endocrinol.* 10, 455-465.

Perez-Gomez, A., et al., 2018. "A Phenotypic *Caenorhabditis elegans* Screen Identifies a Selective Suppressor of Antipsychotic-Induced Hyperphagia." *Nat Commun.* 9, 5272.

Pinto, L.C., Bertoluci, M.C., 2020. "Type 2 Diabetes as a Major Risk Factor for COVID-19 Severity: A Meta-Analysis." *Arch Endocrinol Metab.* 64, 199-200.

Ryu, D., et al., 2016. "Urolithin A Induces Mitophagy and Prolongs Lifespan in *C. elegans* and Increases Muscle Function in Rodents." *Nat Med.* 22, 879-88.

Thaler, J.P., et al., 2012. "Obesity Is Associated with Hypothalamic Injury in Rodents and Humans." *J Clin Invest.* 122, 153-62.

Zhang, Q., Deng, C., Huang, X.F., 2013. "The Role of Ghrelin Signalling in Second-Generation Antipsychotic-Induced Weight Gain." *Psychoneuroendocrinology.* 38, 2423-38.

Made in the USA
Middletown, DE
04 November 2026

36546088R00186